Patient Pictures

Gynaecology

by
Michael Stafford MRCOG
Lecturer/Senior Registrar, Charing Cross and Westminster Medical
School, Chelsea and Westminster Hospital, London, UK

Series Editor
J Richard Smith MD MRCOG
Senior Lecturer and Honorary Consultant Gynaecologist,
Charing Cross and Westminster Medical School,
Chelsea and Westminster Hospital, London, UK

Illustrated by
Dee McLean, MeDee Art, London, UK

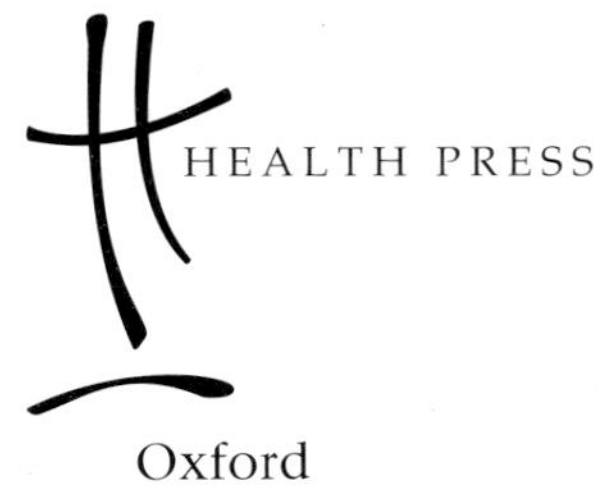

HEALTH PRESS

Oxford

Patient Pictures – Gynaecology

First published 1996

Reprinted 1998

© 1997 Health Press Limited

Elizabeth House, Queen Street, Abingdon, Oxford, UK OX14 3JR

The information herein represents the independent opinion of the author and does not necessarily reflect the opinions and recommendations of Zeneca Pharmaceuticals or the publisher.

A CIP catalogue record for this title is available from the British Library.

ISBN 1-899541-60-8

Typeset by Impressions Design & DTP, Bicester, UK

Designed by Design Online, Oxford, UK

Printed by Uniskill, Witney, UK

Contents

Author's preface

At some stage in their lives, most women will attend a gynaecology clinic, and will want to know how and why a particular disease is affecting them, and what treatments are available. Rather than simply playing a passive role and allowing the doctor 'to do what he thinks best', women now want to be actively involved in the decision-making process regarding their treatment.

This book is intended for healthcare professionals to use with their patients to help achieve this goal. The labelled diagrams, in conjunction with the notes, will help women to understand their anatomy and will explain how a particular operation or procedure works.

Hopefully, this book will also answer many of the concerns women have and, in a small way, help to alleviate anxiety. It should enable women to work with their doctors and make an informed judgement about the best way forward for their healthcare.

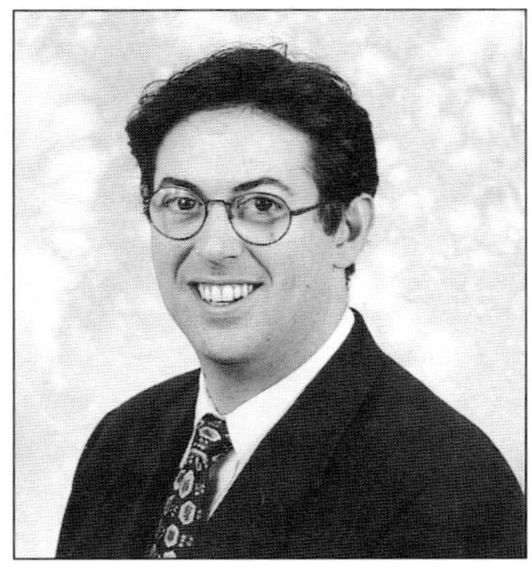

Michael Stafford MRCOG
Lecturer/Senior Registrar
Charing Cross and
Westminster Medical School
Chelsea and Westminster Hospital
London, UK

Reproduction authorization

The purchaser of this *Patient Pictures* series title is hereby authorized
to reproduce by photocopy only, any part of the pictorial and
textual material contained in this work for non-profit, educational,
or patient education use. Photocopying for these purposes only is
welcomed and free from further permission requirements
from the publisher and free from any fee.

The reproduction of any material from this publication outside the
guidelines above is strictly prohibited without the permission in
writing of the publisher and is subject to minimum charges laid
down by the Publishers Licensing Society Limited
or its nominees.

Signed *Sarah Redston* Publisher
Health Press Limited
Oxford

The publisher and the authors have made every effort to ensure the
accuracy of this book, but cannot accept responsibility for
any errors or omissions.

The female genital tract

- The female genital tract includes the vulva, vagina, cervix, uterus, Fallopian tubes and ovaries.

- The vulva is the fleshy folds that surround the opening to the vagina.

- The vagina is a muscular canal or 'tube' which lies between the vulva and the cervix.

- The cervix is a 'barrel-shaped' organ which lies at the end of the vagina. It is sometimes called the 'neck of the womb'.

- The uterus (or womb) extends from the cervix and lies within the pelvis. The uterus is the organ in which the baby develops.

- The endometrium lines the uterus. This lining becomes progressively thicker towards the end of the menstrual cycle in preparation for the fertilized egg. If fertilization does not occur, the top layer of the endometrium breaks down and is lost during menstruation.

- The Fallopian tubes connect the uterus to the ovaries. When an egg is released by an ovary, it passes into the Fallopian tube, where it is fertilized, and then down into the uterus.

- The ovaries lie at the end of each Fallopian tube. Every month, an egg is produced from one of the ovaries and develops in a small 'cyst' (or follicle).

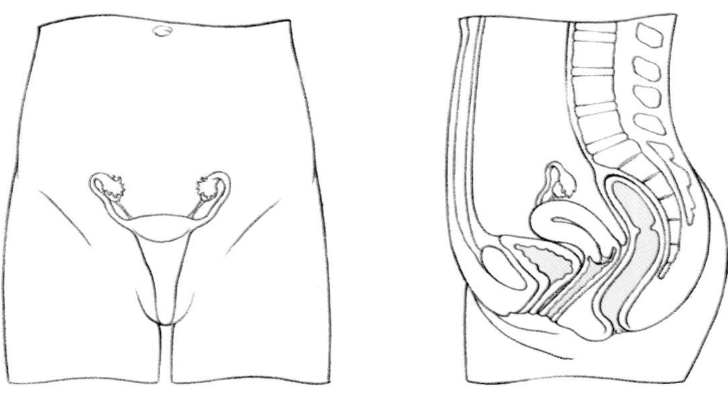

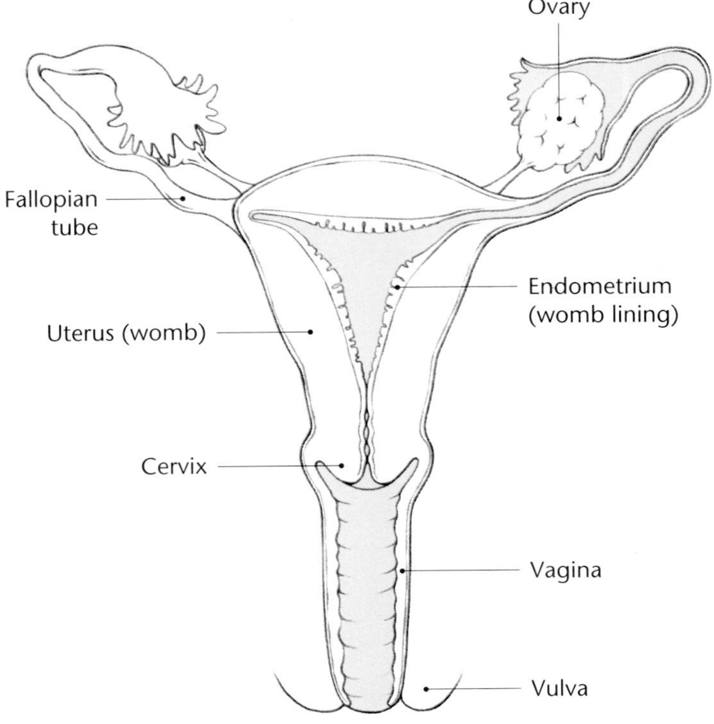

Ovary
Fallopian tube
Endometrium (womb lining)
Uterus (womb)
Cervix
Vagina
Vulva

Position of the uterus

- In 75% of women, the uterus lies forwards towards the pubic bone and is said to be 'anteverted'. In the remaining 25% of women, the uterus lies backwards and is said to be 'retroverted'.

- Certain conditions, such as endometriosis, can cause a uterus that is normally anteverted to become retroverted, which may cause pelvic pain. Very occasionally, an operation may be necessary to correct this.

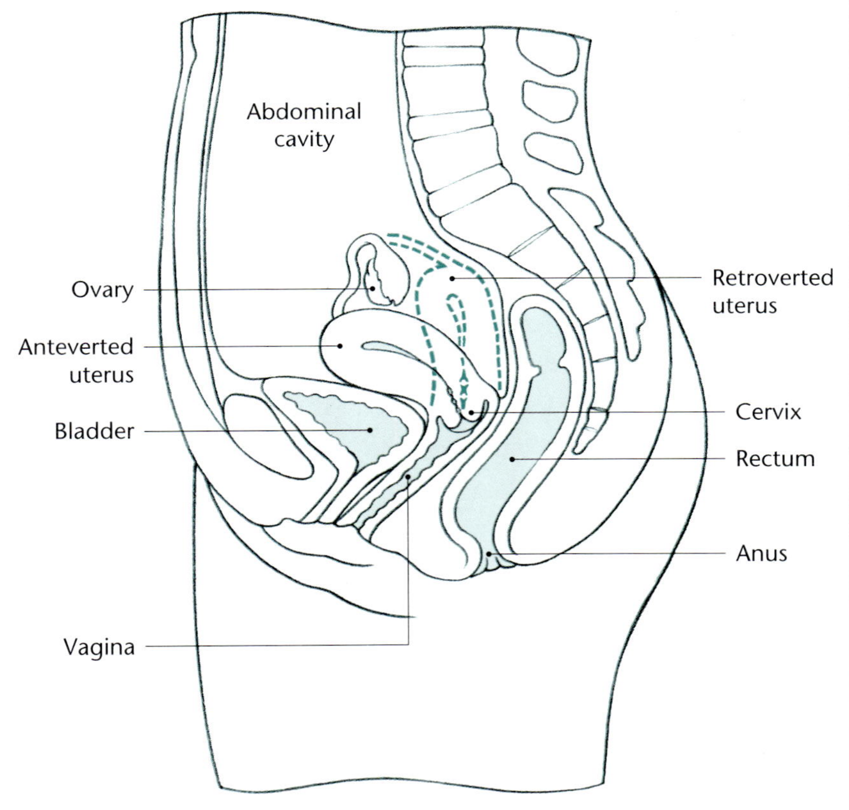

Abdominal cavity
Ovary
Anteverted uterus
Bladder
Vagina
Retroverted uterus
Cervix
Rectum
Anus

Laparoscopy and hysteroscopy

- Laparoscopy is used to examine the abdomen to investigate pelvic pain, ectopic pregnancy and infertility. Hysteroscopy is used to examine the uterus to investigate heavy and/or irregular menstrual bleeding, or postmenopausal bleeding. In both procedures, a small, fibre-optic 'telescope' is used to see the internal organs.

- Both laparoscopy and hysteroscopy are usually performed under a general anaesthetic as a day-case procedure and take 15–20 minutes. Hysteroscopy can also be performed under local anaesthetic as, much more rarely, can laparoscopy.

- In laparoscopy, the instrument is passed through a small incision in the abdomen. A second incision may be made so that a probe can be inserted to manipulate the organs. Carbon dioxide gas is then pumped into the abdomen to separate the tissues so that the organs can be seen more clearly.

- In hysteroscopy, the instrument is passed along the vagina and through the cervix in order to examine the lining of the uterus. No incision is made.

- Patients usually recover from hysteroscopy rapidly. Following laparoscopy, however, patients may experience a pain similar to a period pain or 'wind' for up to 1 week.

- Minimally invasive or 'key-hole' surgery can be performed using laparoscopy and hysteroscopy. This has the advantages of reduced postoperative pain, a shorter hospital stay, a smaller incision and therefore a better cosmetic result than conventional surgery.

LAPAROSCOPY

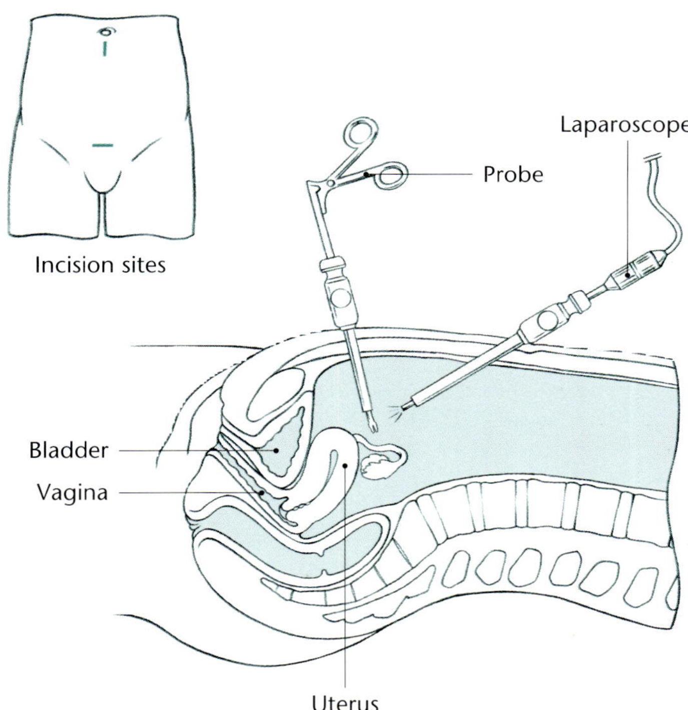

HYSTEROSCOPY

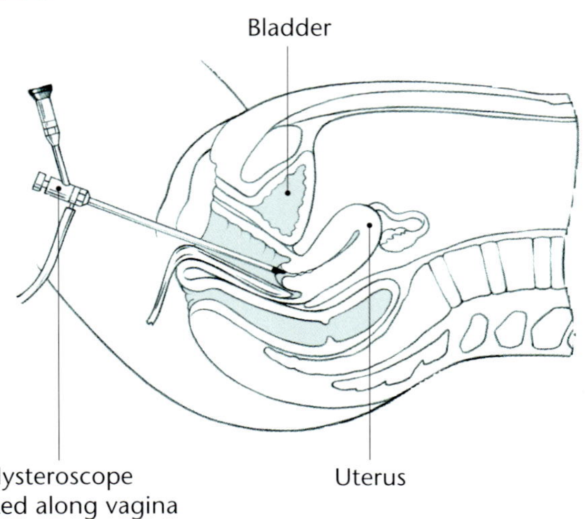

Dilatation and curettage (D & C or uterine evacuation)

- Dilatation and curettage (D & C) may be necessary to investigate abnormal, heavy or irregular bleeding, or to remove what are called the 'products of conception' following miscarriage.

- Nowadays, a hysteroscopy to examine the lining of the uterus is often carried out before a D & C. This involves passing a small, fibre-optic 'telescope' along the vagina and through the cervix in order to examine the lining of the uterus.

- D & C is usually performed under a general anaesthetic as a day-case procedure and takes about 15 minutes.

- The cervix is dilated with a smooth instrument called a dilator. A curette, which is a small, spoon-shaped instrument, is then passed through the cervix to remove the tissue lining the uterus (the endometrium). The tissue is then sent to the laboratory to be examined.

- Patients usually recover rapidly, but may experience discomfort similar to a period pain for a few hours after the procedure. There may also be a small amount of bleeding, which may last 1–2 days.

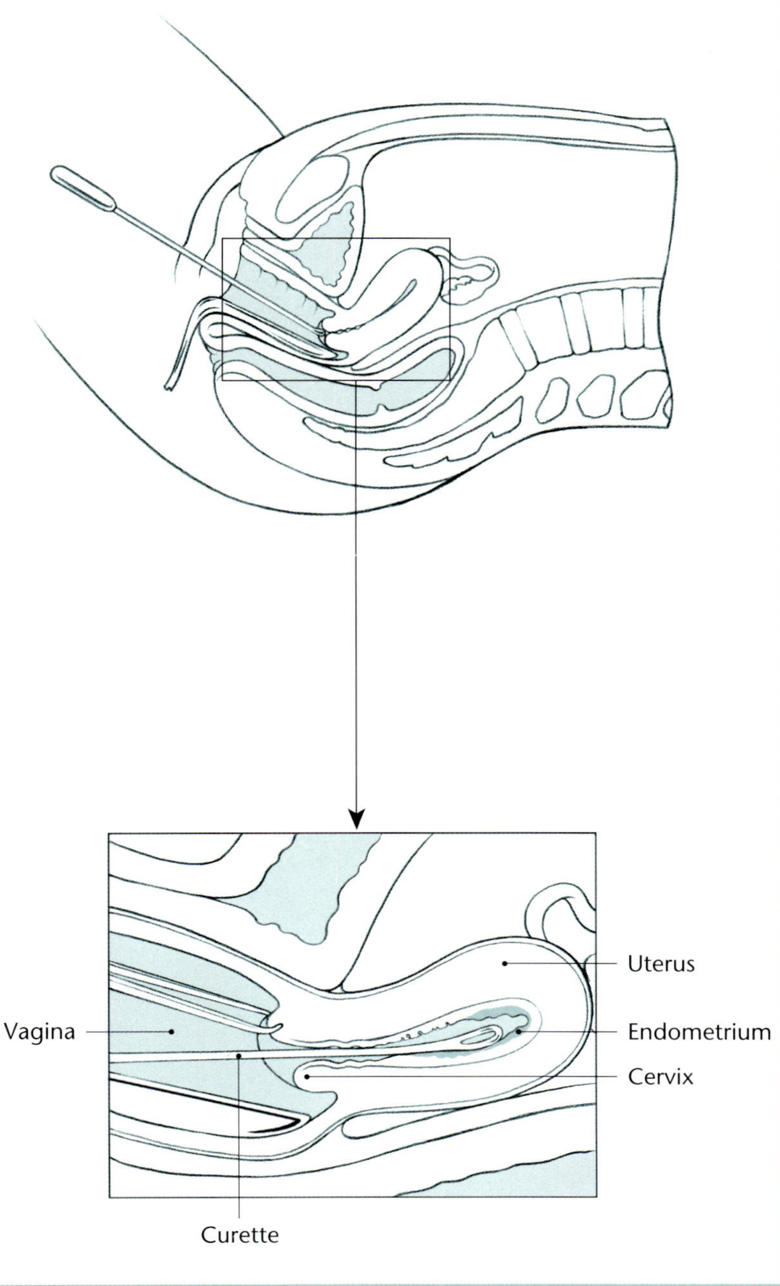

Uterus
Vagina
Endometrium
Cervix
Curette

Cystoscopy

- Cystoscopy is examination of the lining of the bladder using a thin, fibre-optic 'telescope'.

- The procedure is used to investigate the cause of urinary symptoms, such as urgency, frequency or blood in the urine, or as part of the investigation of cancer of the cervix.

- Cystoscopy is usually performed under a general anaesthetic as a day-case procedure and takes about 5–10 minutes.

- The urethra (the tube through which urine passes from the bladder to the outside) is dilated and the bladder filled with fluid through a soft plastic tube called a catheter. The cystoscope is then inserted to examine the lining of the bladder.

- Normal activities can be resumed the following day.

- In patients undergoing major abdominal surgery (e.g. for cancer of the cervix or ovary), cystoscopy may be used to insert plastic stents into the ureters (the tubes which drain the urine from the kidneys into the bladder), so that the surgeon can identify them more easily. The stents are removed after surgery.

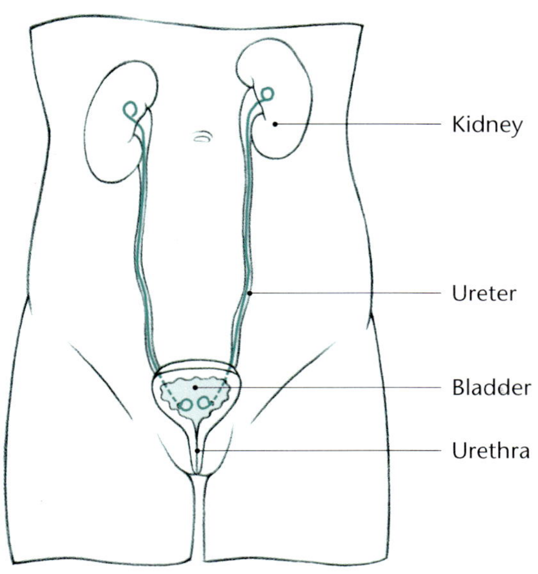

Kidney
Ureter
Bladder
Urethra

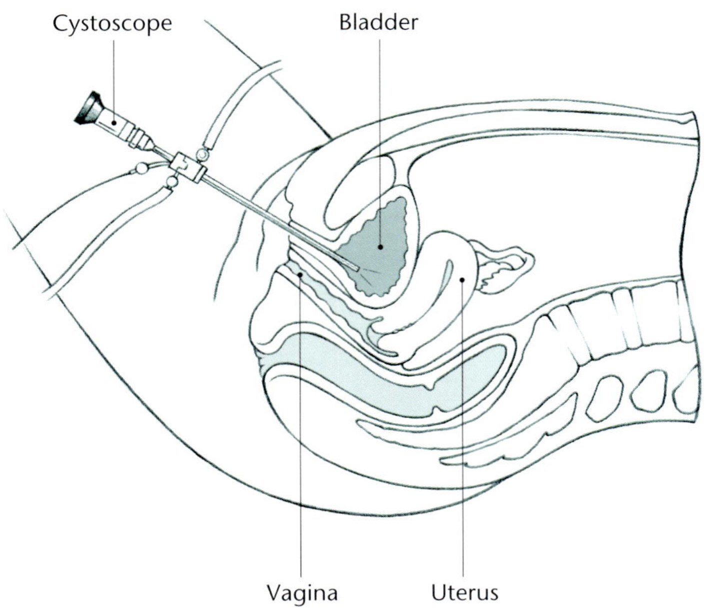

Cystoscope
Bladder
Vagina
Uterus

Hysterectomy – total and subtotal

- Hysterectomy is used to treat menstrual problems and chronic pelvic pain caused by endometriosis and pelvic inflammatory disease (PID).

- A total hysterectomy involves removal of the uterus and the cervix. The vagina is closed over at the top and remains the normal length.

- A subtotal hysterectomy involves removal of the uterus only. The cervix is left intact and the vagina remains the normal length. This operation is performed only if a woman wishes to keep her cervix or if there are technical difficulties with the operation.

- The operation is performed under a general anaesthetic and takes about 1 hour.

- During the operation, a catheter will be passed up the urethra into the bladder to drain off the urine. A plastic tube may also be inserted into the wound to remove any slight bleeding. These tubes will be left in place for 24–48 hours.

- Although there will be some discomfort following surgery, this will be controlled with pain killers.

- The average length of stay in hospital is 5–7 days and normal activities can be resumed within 6–8 weeks.

- There should be no problems with sexual intercourse following the operation.

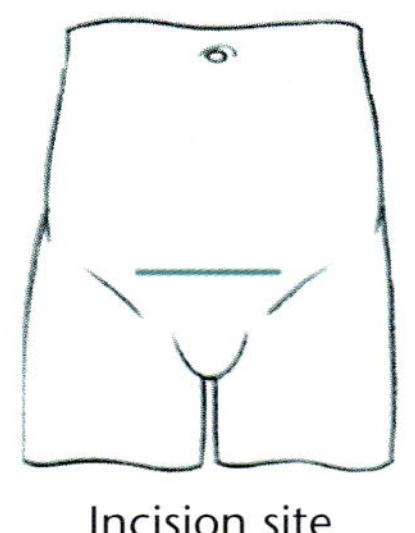

Incision site

TOTAL HYSTERECTOMY

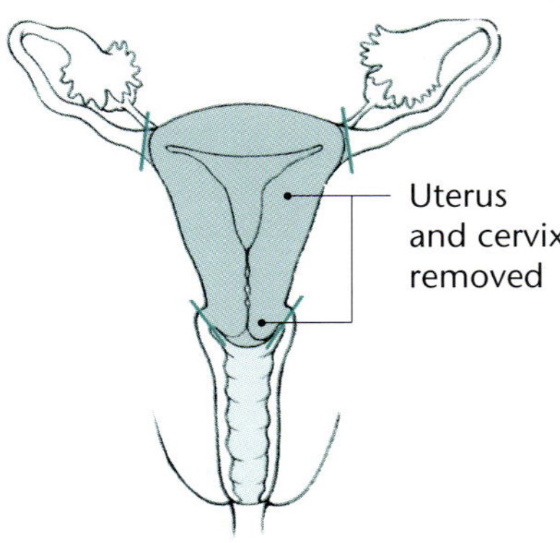

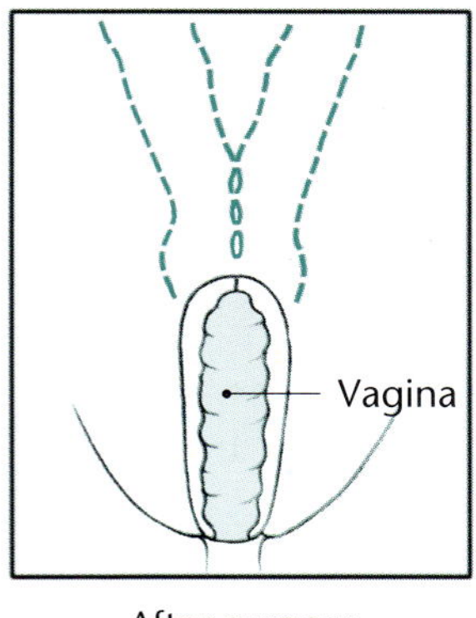

After surgery

SUBTOTAL HYSTERECTOMY

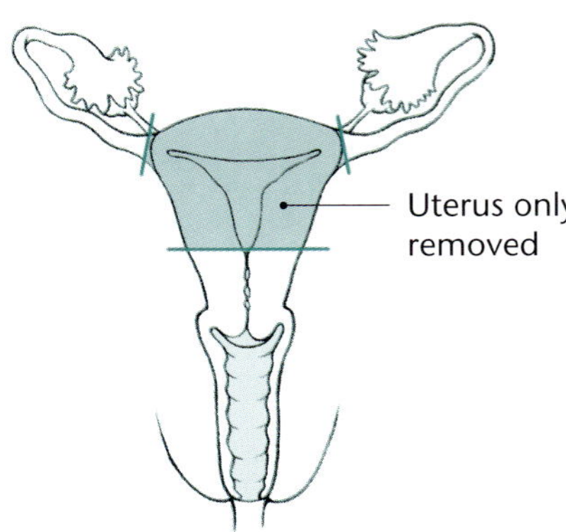

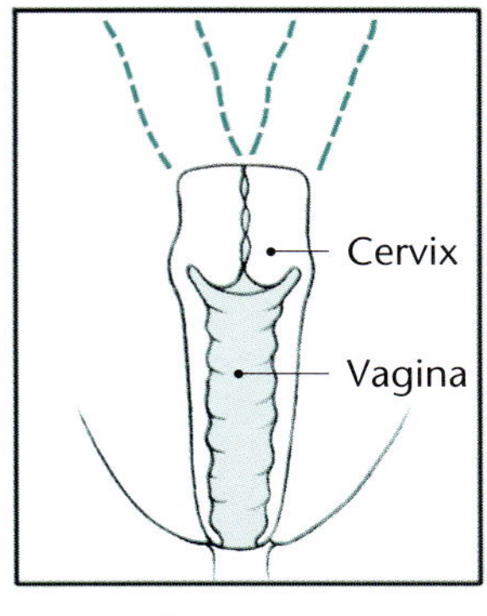

After surgery

Hysterectomy and bilateral salpingo-oophorectomy

- A hysterectomy can be used to treat menstrual problems in women approaching the menopause. Bilateral salpingo-oophorectomy, which is removal of the ovaries, is carried out to prevent the risk of ovarian cancer in the future and the formation of scar tissue which may cause long-term pain.

- The two procedures are carried out in one operation, which involves the removal of the uterus, Fallopian tubes, cervix and ovaries. The vagina is closed over at the top and remains the normal length.

- The operation is performed under a general anaesthetic and takes about 1 hour.

- During the operation, a catheter will be passed up the urethra into the bladder to drain off the urine. A plastic tube may also be inserted into the wound to remove any slight bleeding. These tubes will be left in place for 24–48 hours.

- Although there will be some discomfort following surgery, this will be controlled with pain killers.

- The average length of stay in hospital is 5–7 days and normal activities can be resumed within 6–8 weeks.

- Hormone replacement therapy (HRT) may be prescribed to replace the ovarian hormones, depending upon the age of the patient.

- There should be no problems with sexual intercourse following the operation.

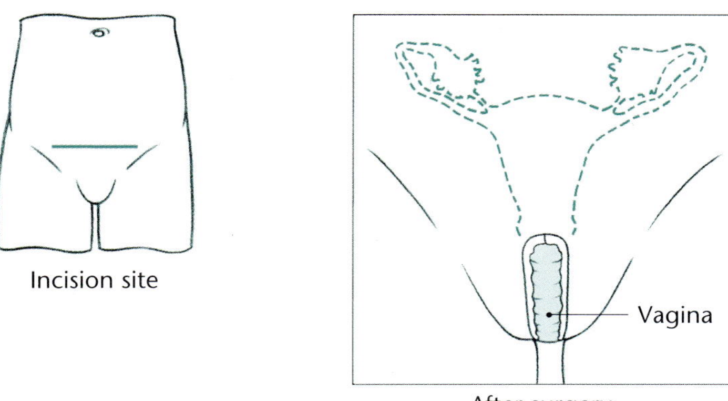
Incision site
Vagina
After surgery

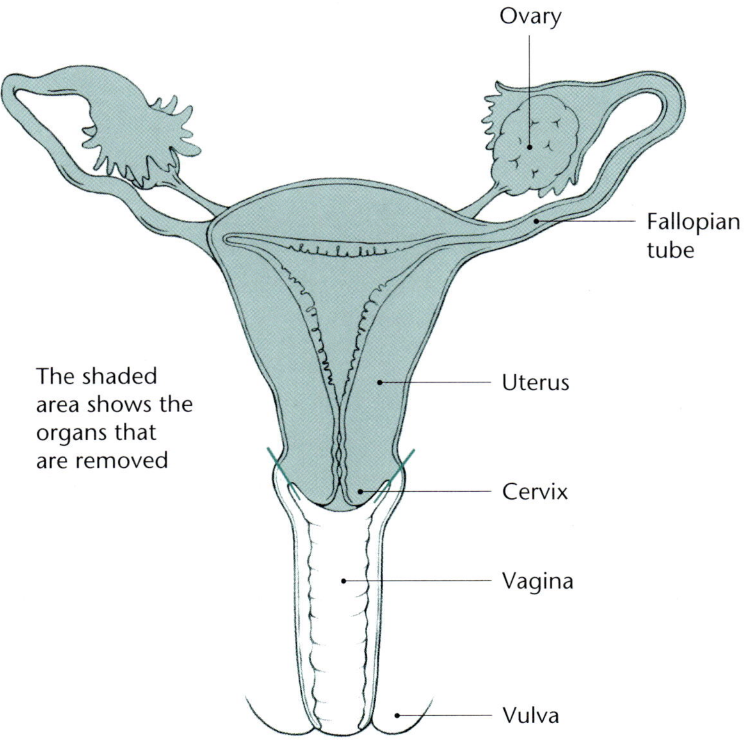
Ovary
Fallopian tube
The shaded area shows the organs that are removed
Uterus
Cervix
Vagina
Vulva

Myomectomy

- Myomectomy involves the removal of uterine fibroids. The uterus, cervix, Fallopian tubes, ovaries and vagina all remain intact.

- Fibroids are lumps which form in the wall of the uterus. They can cause heavy menstrual bleeding and are occasionally painful, especially in pregnancy. Fibroids occur for no apparent reason, and are completely non-cancerous.

- The operation is performed under a general anaesthetic, and the time taken will depend on the number and size of the fibroids to be removed, but is usually 1–2 hours.

- During the operation, a catheter may be passed up the urethra into the bladder to drain off the urine. A plastic tube may also be inserted into the wound to remove any slight bleeding. These tubes will be left in place for 24–48 hours.

- There is a small chance that a hysterectomy may be needed, if any bleeding cannot be stopped.

- Patients may develop a temperature immediately after the operation, but this is quite normal. Although there will be some discomfort following surgery, this will be controlled with pain killers. Vaginal bleeding may also occur, but is usually light.

- The average length of stay in hospital is 5–7 days and normal activities can be resumed within 6–8 weeks.

- There should be no problems with sexual intercourse following the operation.

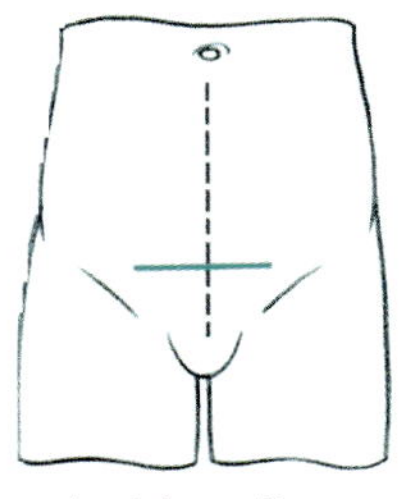

Incision sites
small fibroids
large fibroids

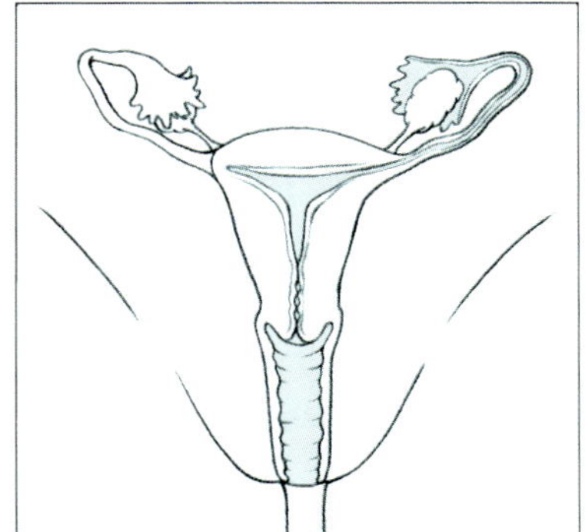

After surgery

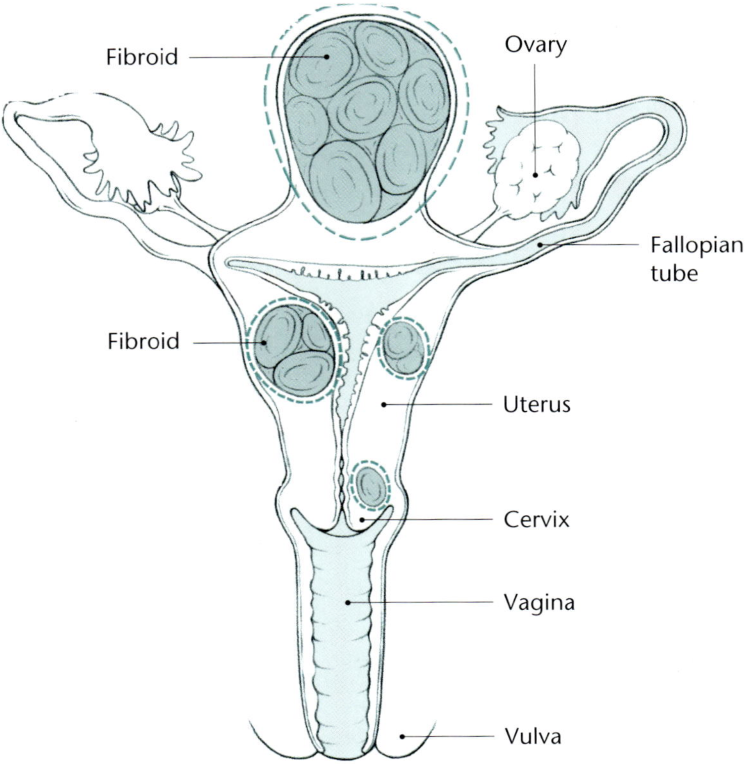

Fibroid
Ovary
Fallopian tube
Fibroid
Uterus
Cervix
Vagina
Vulva

Endometrial ablation

- Endometrial ablation is an alternative to hysterectomy as a treatment for menstrual bleeding problems. The procedure involves stripping the lining of the uterus so that the tissue which produces the menstrual bleeding is destroyed or 'ablated'.

- Hormonal drugs may need to be taken for a period before the operation in order to 'thin' the lining of the uterus, and make the operation easier and more successful.

- The operation is performed under a general anaesthetic and takes about 1 hour.

- The cervix is dilated to allow a fibre-optic 'telescope' called an hysteroscope to be inserted into the uterus so that the lining can be seen.

- The tissue lining the uterus can then be destroyed by a laser, or stripped away using a hot, wire loop called a resectoscope or a heated revolving ball.

- After the operation, pain killers may be necessary and some light bleeding may occur.

- The average hospital stay is 24–48 hours and normal activities can usually be resumed in 2–3 weeks.

- Menstrual periods may not be entirely abolished following this procedure: 25% of women have no periods; 40–50% have acceptable periods; and 25% find the operation unhelpful in the long term.

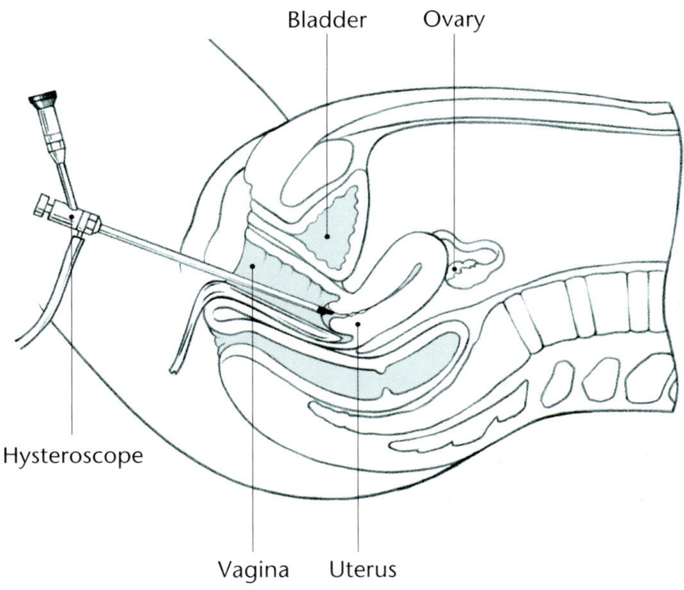

Bladder
Ovary
Hysteroscope
Vagina
Uterus

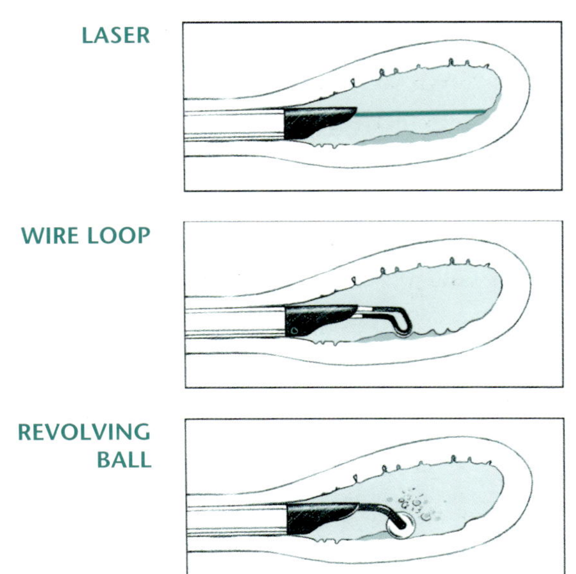

LASER
WIRE LOOP
REVOLVING
BALL

Salpingectomy

- Salpingectomy is usually necessary because of previous pelvic inflammatory disease (PID) or to remove an ectopic pregnancy. It involves partial or total removal of a Fallopian tube. The uterus and ovaries are left intact.

- The operation is performed under a general anaesthetic and takes 30–60 minutes. It is sometimes performed as an emergency.

- The procedure is commonly performed laparoscopically, using a small, fibre-optic 'telescope' which is inserted into the abdomen through a small incision. Occasionally a conventional operation (laparotomy) is used.

- There will be some discomfort following surgery which will be controlled with pain killers.

- The average hospital stay is 2–6 days and will depend on the type of surgery. Complete recovery should occur within 6 weeks.

- Women who have both Fallopian tubes removed will only be able to become pregnant by *in vitro* fertilization (IVF).

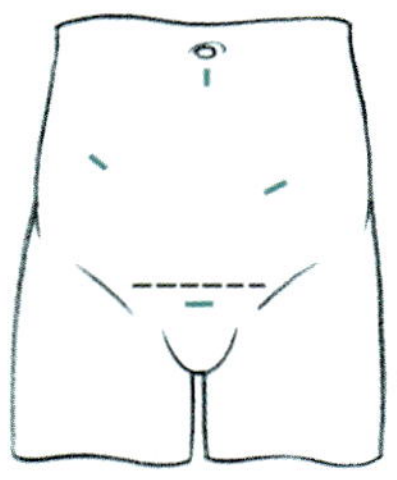

Incision sites
— for laparoscopy
---- for laparotomy

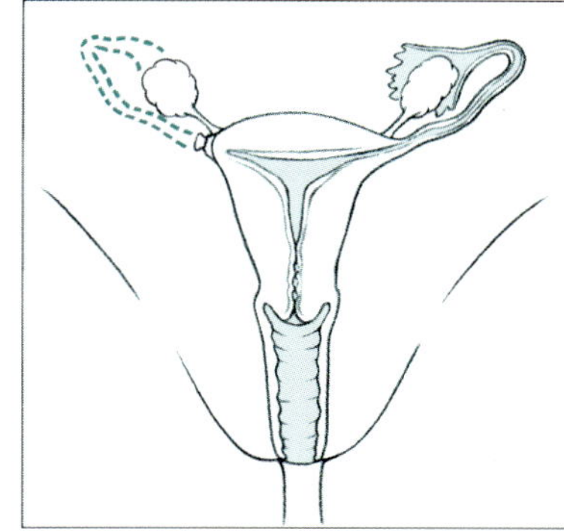

After surgery

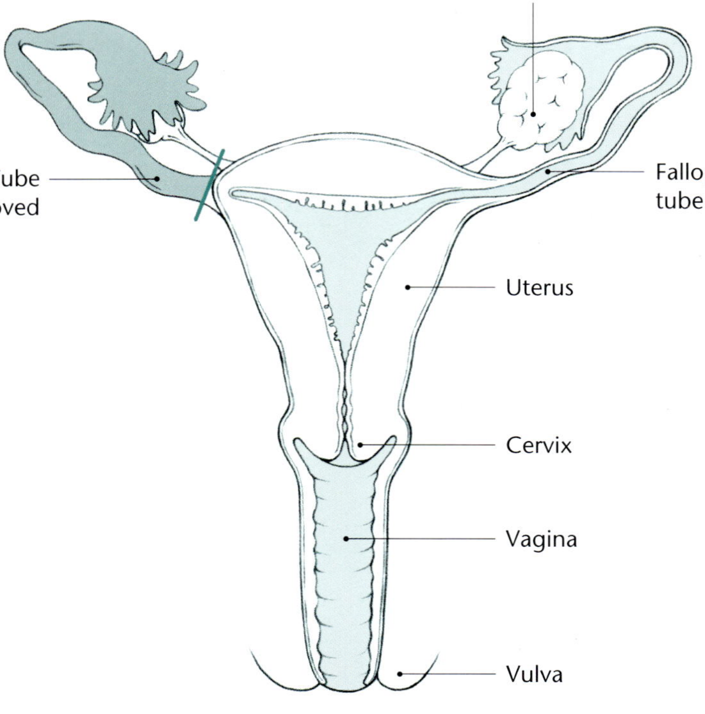

Ovary
Tube removed
Fallopian tube
Uterus
Cervix
Vagina
Vulva

Salpingostomy

- A salpingostomy is used to treat infertility caused by blockage of the Fallopian tube. This blockage is usually a result of a previous infection.

- The operation is performed under a general anaesthetic and takes about 1 hour.

- The procedure is commonly performed laparoscopically, using a small, fibre-optic 'telescope' which is inserted into the abdomen through a small incision. Occasionally a conventional operation (laparotomy) is used.

- Incisions are made in the end of the tube to release any scar tissue and open the blocked tube. The ovary is not affected.

- There will be some discomfort following surgery which will be controlled with pain killers.

- The average hospital stay is 5–7 days and complete recovery should occur within 6 weeks.

- Generally, the tubes can be opened successfully in 90% of women, and 60–80% will subsequently become pregnant.

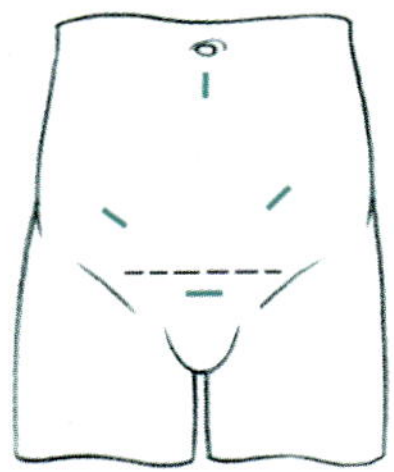

Incision sites
— for laparoscopy
---- for laparotomy

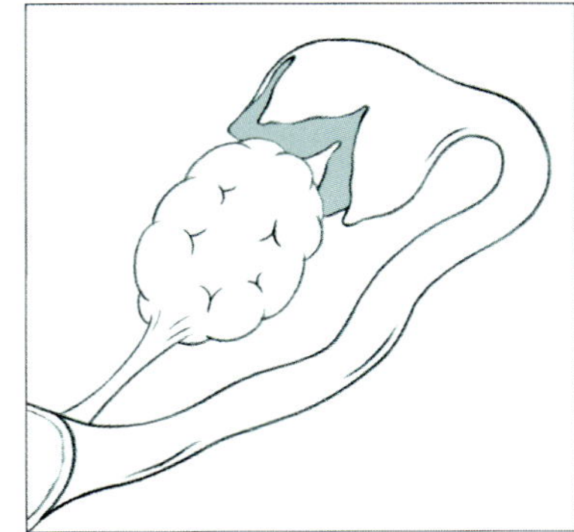

After surgery – the
Fallopian tube is open

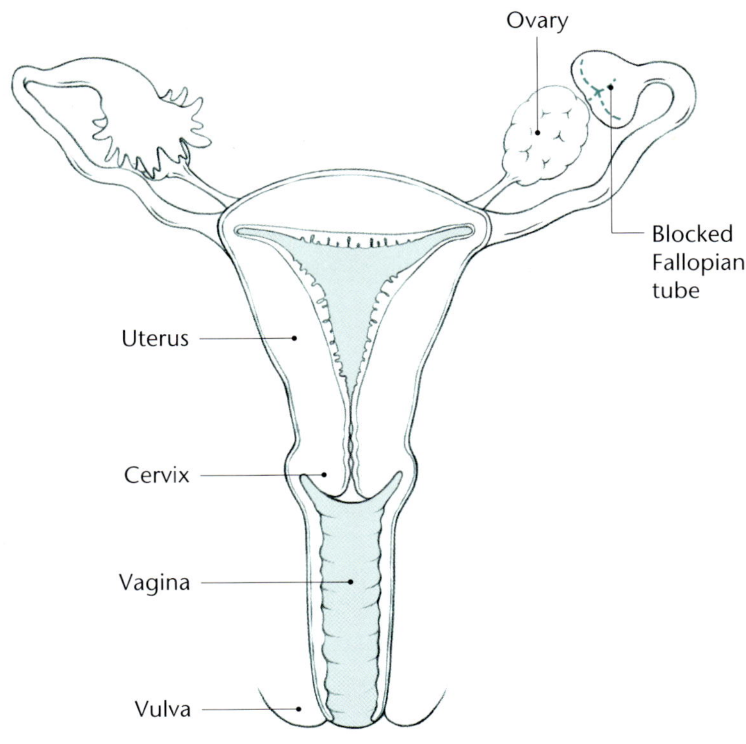

Laparoscopic adhesiolysis

- Laparoscopic adhesiolysis is used to remove scar tissue called adhesions, which are caused by infection or previous surgery in patients with chronic pelvic pain or infertility. As a result of this scar tissue, organs which are normally separate, such as the bladder and bowel, can become 'stuck' together causing pain.

- The operation is performed under a general anaesthetic, and the length of time taken will vary from 30 minutes to 2 hours depending on the number of adhesions.

- The procedure is performed laparoscopically, using a small, fibre-optic 'telescope', which is inserted into the abdomen through a small incision. The adhesions are broken down with specially designed instruments. All the organs remain intact.

- There will be some discomfort following surgery which is controlled with pain killers.

- The average hospital stay is 1–2 days and complete recovery should occur within 2 weeks.

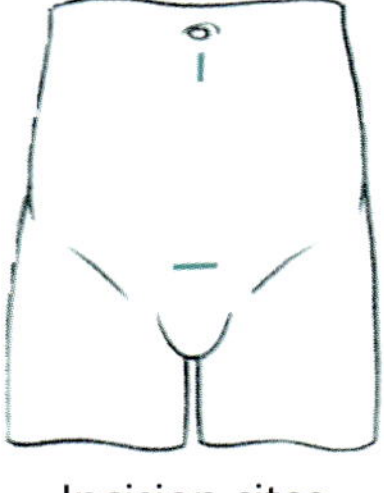

Incision sites

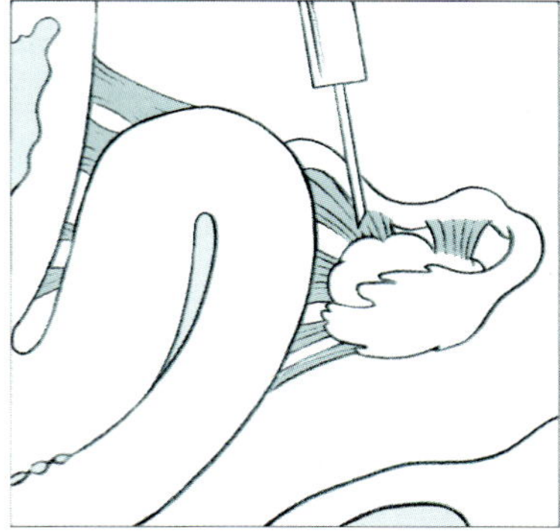

Adhesions being broken down

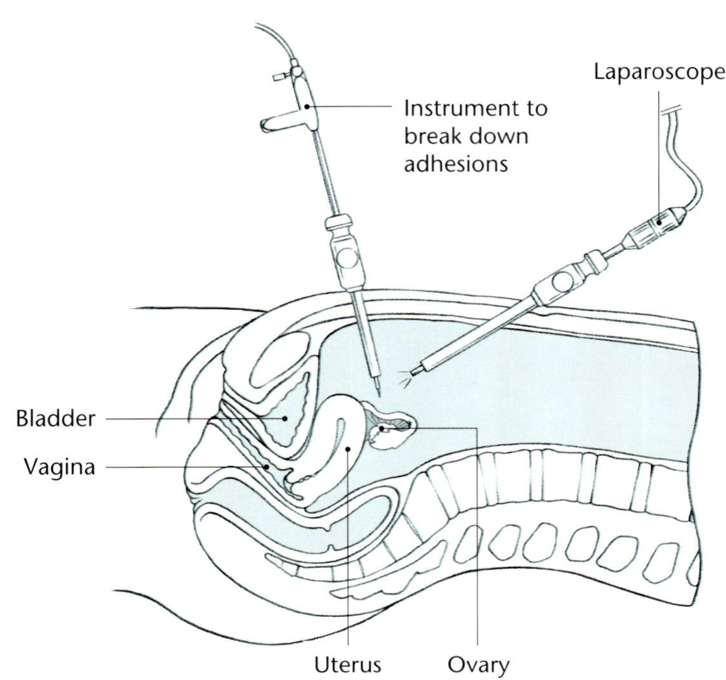

Removal of ectopic pregnancy

- A pregnancy which occurs in the Fallopian tube is called ectopic. This must be removed to prevent excessive bleeding which may result if the tube ruptures.

- The operation may involve removal of the tube and pregnancy (salpingectomy), or removal of the pregnancy only (linear salpingostomy)

- The operation is performed as an emergency procedure under a general anaesthetic and takes 30–60 minutes.

- The procedure is commonly performed laparoscopically, using a small, fibre-optic 'telescope' which is inserted into the abdomen through a small incision. Occasionally, a conventional operation (laparotomy) is used.

- There will be some discomfort following surgery which will be controlled with pain killers.

- The average hospital stay is 2–6 days and will depend on the type of surgery. Complete recovery should occur within 6 weeks.

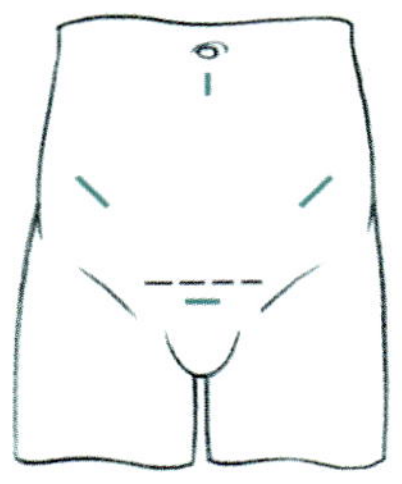

Incision sites
—— for laparoscopy
---- for laparotomy

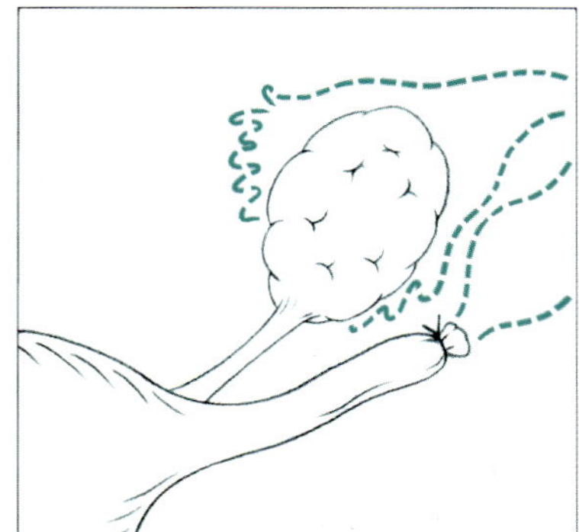

After surgery

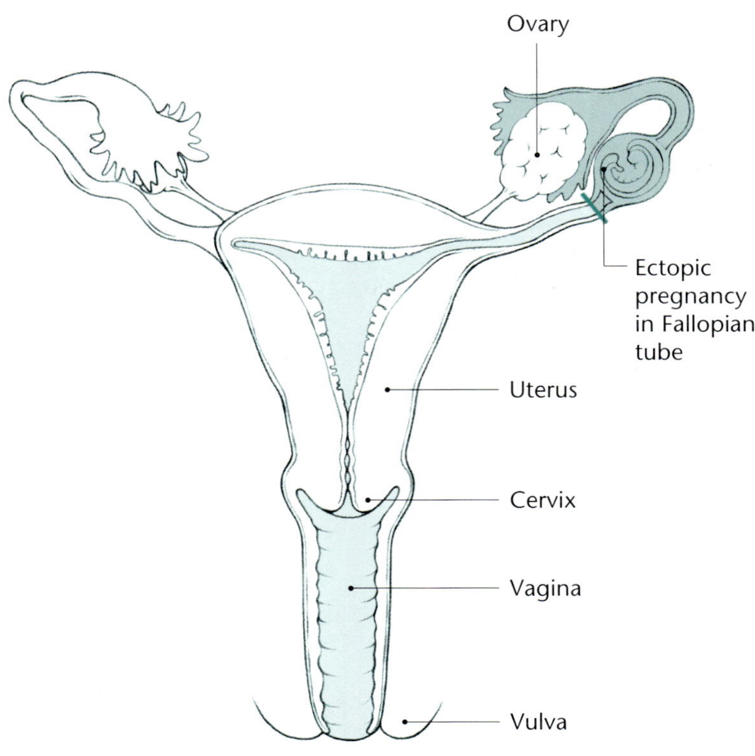

Oophorectomy

- Oophorectomy is the removal of one or both ovaries, which may be necessary because of ovarian cysts or ovarian pain. The uterus is left intact.

- The operation is performed under a general anaesthetic and takes about 1 hour.

- The procedure is commonly performed laparoscopically, using a small, fibre-optic 'telescope' which is inserted into the abdomen through a small incision. Occasionally a conventional operation (laparotomy) is used.

- There will be some discomfort following surgery, which will be controlled with pain killers.

- The average length of stay in hospital is 48 hours following laparoscopy and 5–7 days following conventional surgery. Complete recovery is quicker following laparoscopy, but usually occurs within 6 weeks.

- If both ovaries are removed, hormone replacement therapy (HRT) will usually be given following surgery.

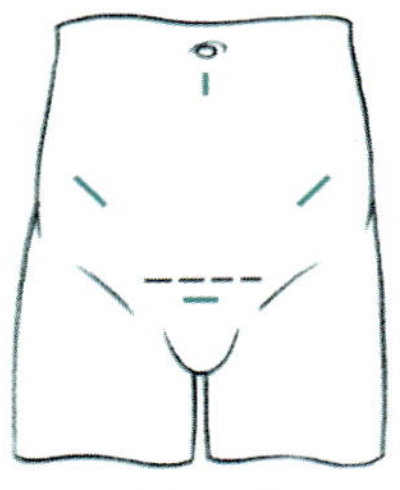

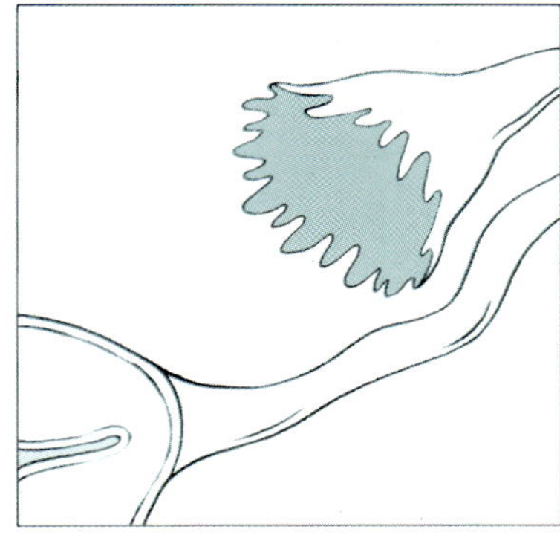

After surgery

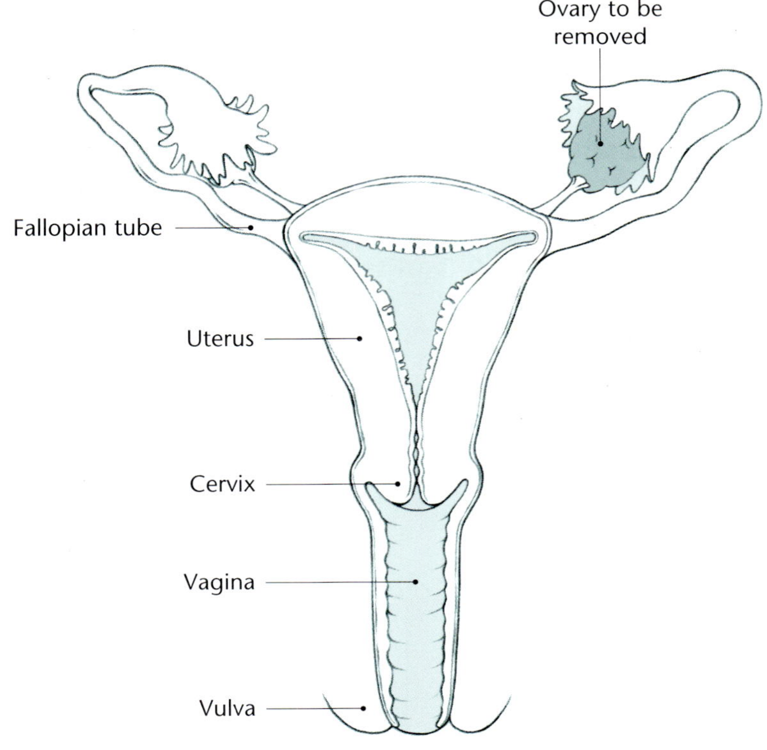

Ovarian cystectomy

- Ovarian cystectomy is performed to remove non-cancerous cysts.

- The operation is carried out under a general anaesthetic and takes about 40–60 minutes.

- The procedure is commonly performed laparoscopically, using a small, fibre-optic 'telescope' which is inserted into the abdomen through a small incision. Occasionally a conventional operation (laparotomy) is used.

- The cyst is carefully cut away from the ovary and sent for laboratory testing. The ovary is then stitched and returned to its normal size and shape. The Fallopian tubes are unaffected.

- There will be some discomfort following surgery which will be controlled with pain killers.

- The ovarian hormone levels are unchanged and fertility should be unaffected.

- The average hospital stay is 5–7 days and complete recovery usually occurs within 6 weeks. If the operation has been performed using 'key-hole' surgery (laparoscopy), the recovery time will be shorter.

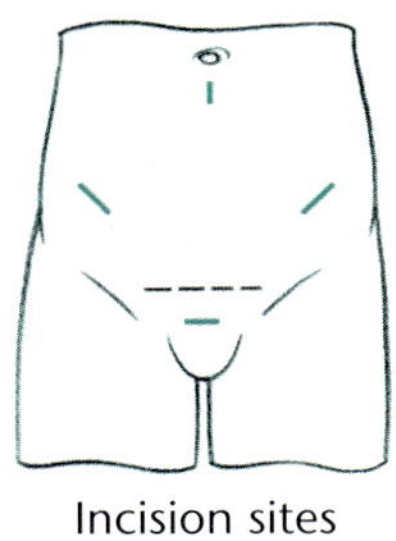

Incision sites
—— for laparoscopy
---- for laparotomy

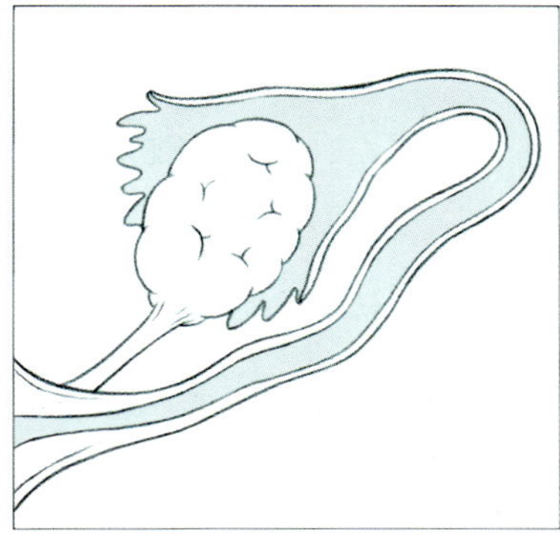

After surgery

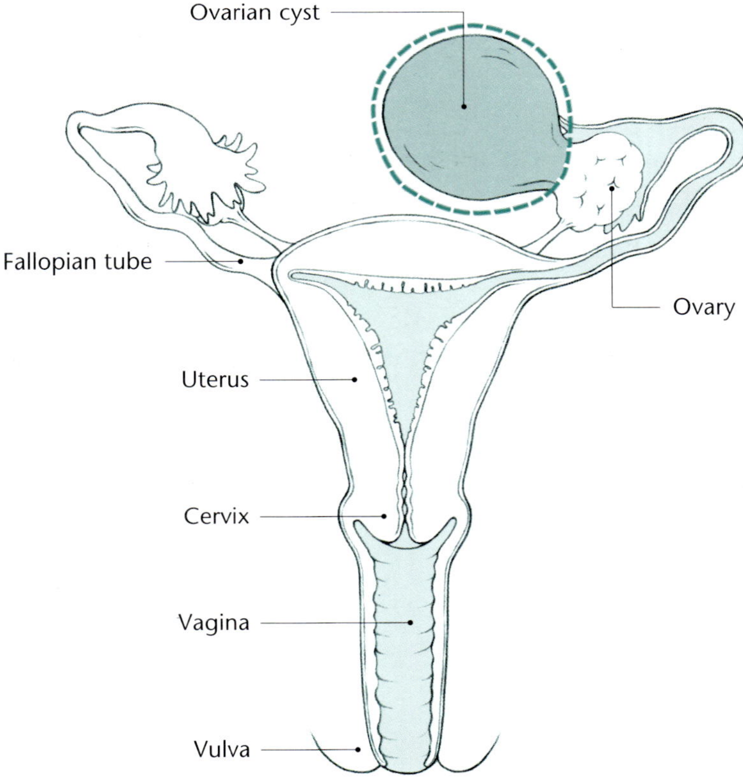

Ovarian cyst
Fallopian tube
Ovary
Uterus
Cervix
Vagina
Vulva

Marsupialization of a Bartholin's cyst or abscess

- The Bartholin's glands lie at the entrance to the vagina and secrete mucus. The duct to a gland can become blocked causing a small swelling called a cyst. If this cyst becomes infected, an abscess containing pus forms.

- A 'marsupialization', which simply means to form a pouch, is performed to allow the mucus secreted by the gland to drain away.

- The operation is performed under a general anaesthetic, sometimes as an emergency procedure, and takes 10–15 minutes.

- During surgery a small 'wick' of cotton gauze will usually be inserted into the cyst cavity to help the gland drain and prevent the cavity from healing over. This 'wick' will be removed the following day.

- There will be some discomfort following surgery which will be controlled with pain killers.

- The average hospital stay is 24–48 hours and normal activities can usually be resumed within 2–3 days.

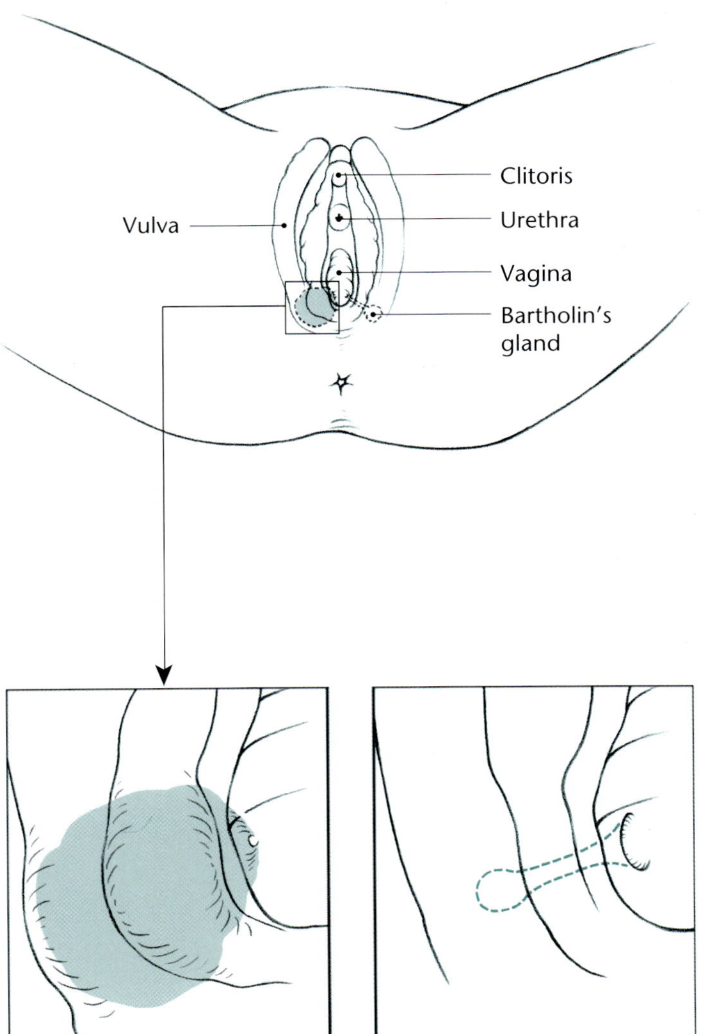

Before surgery, the gland is swollen and possibly infected

After surgery, the gland is restored to normal

Contraception – the options

- The combined oral contraceptive pill, which contains the hormones oestrogen and progestogen, is very effective and must be taken daily. Occasionally, bleeding can occur mid-cycle.

- The progestogen-only or 'mini-pill' is another form of oral contraception and must also be taken daily. 'Spotting' or irregular bleeding can occur.

- Hormone injections contain progestogen only and provide contraception for 12 weeks, after which time another injection must be given.

- Hormone implants contain progestogen only and are effective for 5 years; unlike injections, implants can be removed at any time. Bleeding can, however, be irregular.

- The intrauterine contraceptive device (IUCD) is inserted at a clinic under medical supervision. Periods can be heavy after insertion. The device is usually replaced after 5 years.

- The intrauterine system (IUS) is an intrauterine contraceptive that contains the hormone levonorgestrel. In addition to providing contraception, it also helps to lighten heavy periods.

- The diaphragm and cervical cap are inserted before sexual intercourse. They should both be used in conjunction with a spermicide.

- Sterilization involves an operation. In a woman, this involves closing off the tubes that carry the egg from the ovary to the womb. This form of contraception should be considered permanent.

		Failure rate (number of pregnancies/100 women/year)	
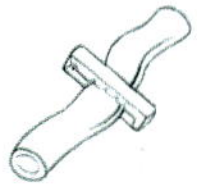	Sterilization	0–0.5	R
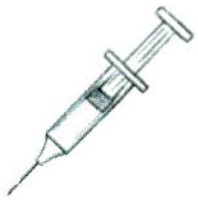	Hormone injection	0–1	E
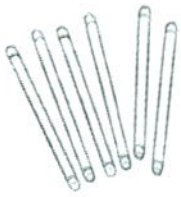	Hormone implant	0–1	L
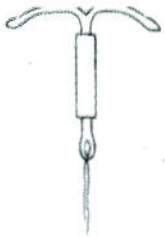	Intrauterine hormone system	0.14	I
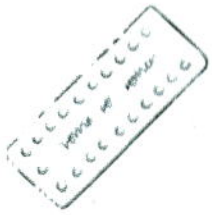	Combined oral contraceptive pill	0.1–3.0	A
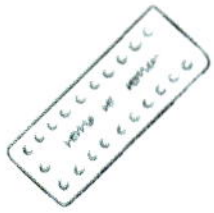	Progestogen-only pill	0.3–4.0	B
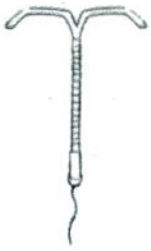	Intrauterine contraceptive device	0.3–2+	I L I T Y
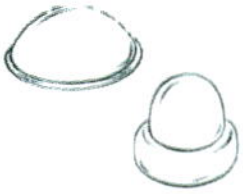	Diaphragm and cervical cap	2–15	
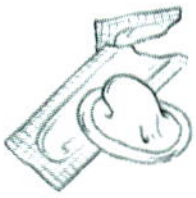	Condoms	2–15	

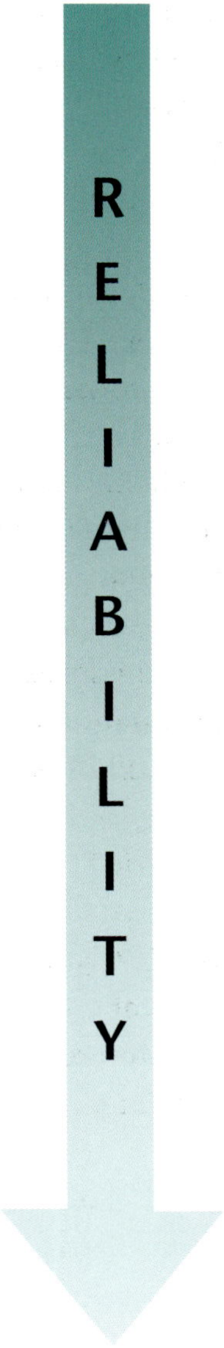

Intrauterine contraceptive device (IUCD)

- The intrauterine contraceptive device (IUCD) is a well-established and reliable form of contraception. It is more often used by women who have had at least one child, because the cervix has been dilated and therefore insertion is easier. It is however, possible for a woman who has had no children to use an IUCD.

- The device is usually inserted immediately following a period. The procedure can usually be carried out at a clinic, without the need for any anaesthetic, and takes 2–3 minutes.

- An instrument called a speculum is inserted to hold the walls of the vagina apart. The IUCD is then placed in the uterus using a fine plastic introducer.

- A string leads from the IUCD through the cervix. This is necessary to aid removal and to allow the woman to check that it is still in position, though it is unlikely to be dislodged.

- The IUCD can, if desired, remain in place for 3–8 years.

- The IUCD has the advantages that there are no worries about remembering to use contraception and it does not interfere with intercourse. The IUCD may, however, cause slightly heavier periods or period pain.

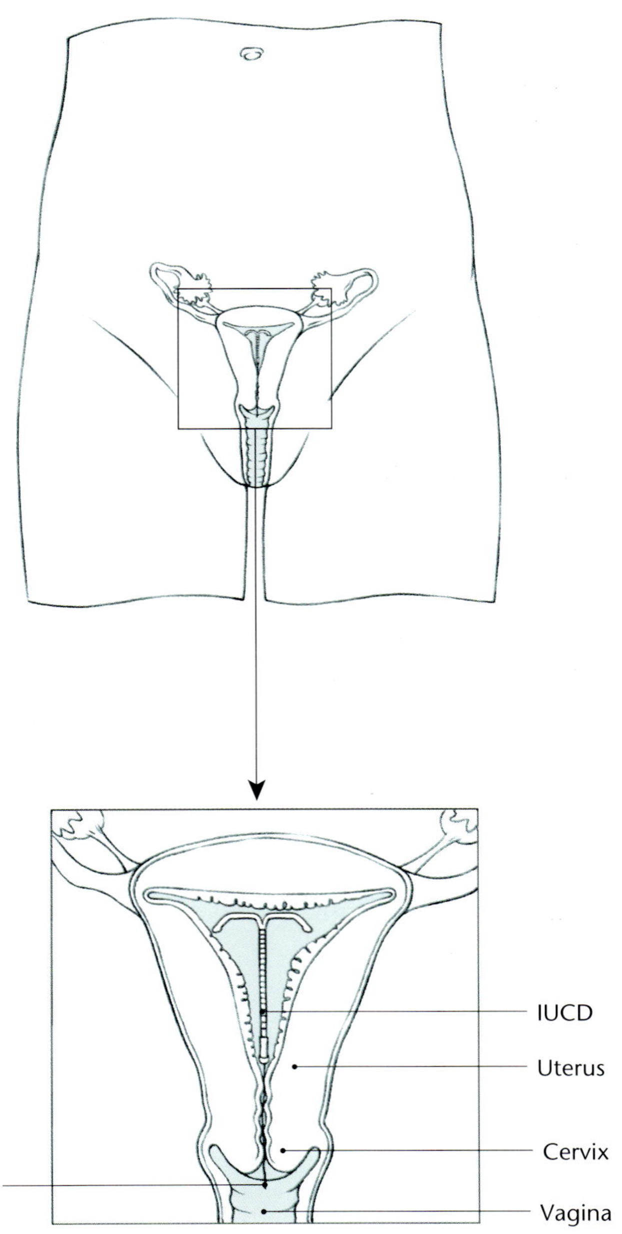

IUCD
Uterus
Cervix
'String'
Vagina

Cervical cap and diaphragm

- The cervical cap and diaphragm are two types of barrier contraception, which prevent the sperm entering the cervix. Both devices are reliable forms of contraception when used with a spermicide.

- The initial fitting is carried out by a trained family planning nurse, who will also give instruction on how to use the device.

- Correct insertion is important. The cap should lie directly over the cervical opening, and the diaphragm across the top of the vagina and over the cervical opening.

- Women using the cervical cap must examine themselves before insertion to establish the position of the cervix. It is important to be aware that cervical position may alter at certain times of the month and throughout life.

- Both the cervical cap and the diaphragm should be left in position for 6 hours after intercourse to ensure that sperm that remain in the vagina do not enter the uterine cavity.

- The cervical cap and diaphragm must be refitted after pregnancy, and after a significant change in weight, because your anatomy can alter.

CERVICAL CAP

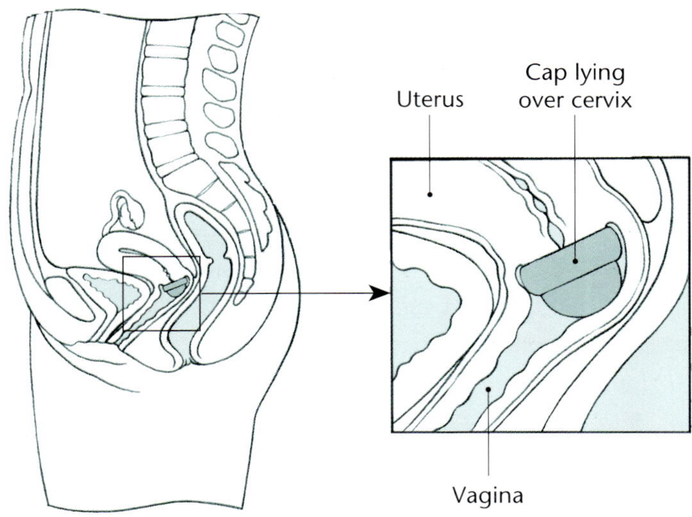

DIAPHRAGM

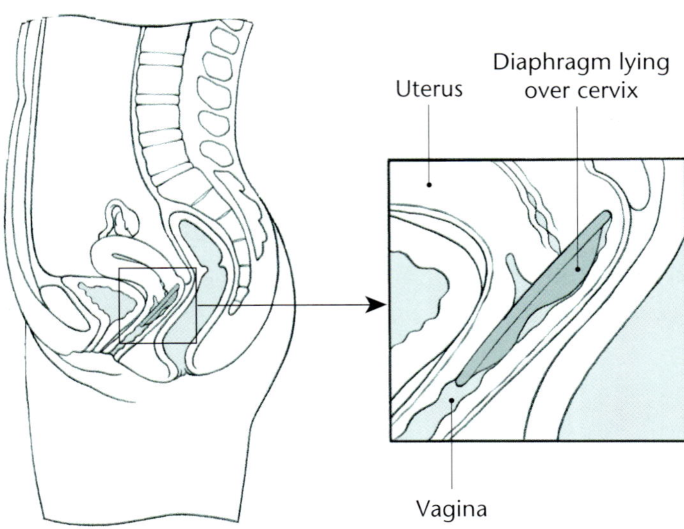

Sterilization

- Sterilization should only be undertaken after careful thought and should be considered irreversible.

- The operation is carried out under general anaesthetic as a day-case procedure.

- A small, fibre-optic 'telescope' called a laparoscope is inserted into the abdomen through a small incision. Carbon dioxide gas is then pumped into the abdomen to separate the tissues so that the organs can be seen more clearly. Plastic clips, which remain in place permanently, are then placed on the Fallopian tubes.

- If the tubes are difficult to see through the laparoscope, it may be necessary to make a slightly larger incision in the abdomen, which will be 2–3 inches in length, in order to complete the procedure successfully.

- Women who have been using the oral contraceptive can stop doing so when they reach the end of the packet. However, menstrual periods will return to the same pattern and type of bleeding as before the pill was used.

- Period type cramps can occur after the operation, but it should be possible to return to normal activities within 48 hours.

- There is a small failure rate (about 1 in 500), but sterilization is considered to be the most reliable form of contraception.

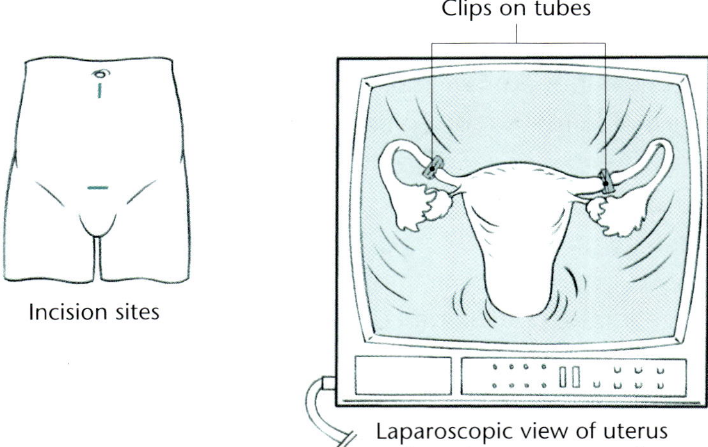

Incision sites

Laparoscopic view of uterus
and ovaries seen on monitor

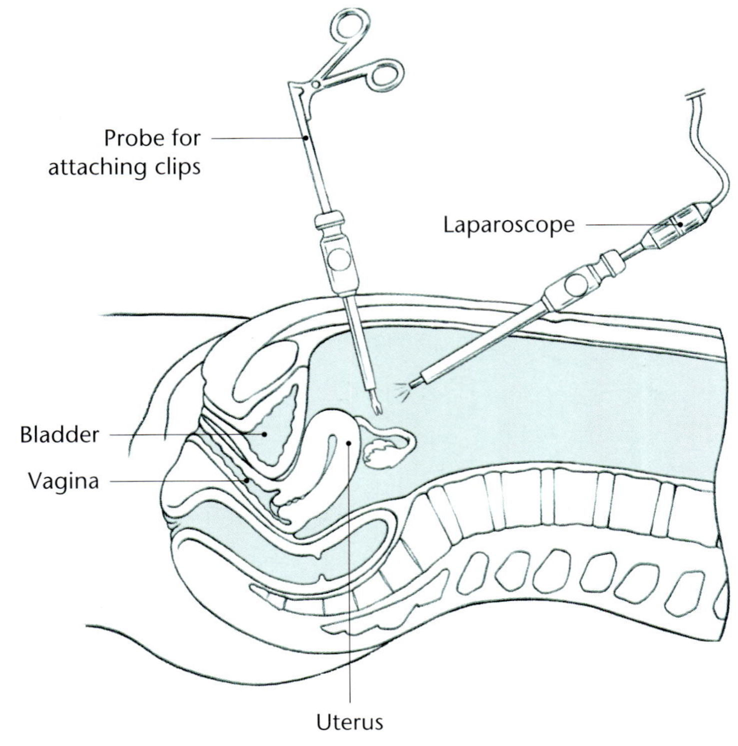

Colposcopy

- A colposcopy is carried out when abnormalities have been seen on a cervical smear. The colposcope is a microscope which magnifies the cervix and enables it to be examined more closely.

- Colposcopy is a painless procedure performed in out-patients. An instrument called a speculum is inserted to hold the walls of the vagina apart and the cervix is then examined with the colposcope.

- Dilute acetic acid and iodine may be painted onto the cervix in order to highlight any abnormal changes.

- Small pieces of tissue called biopsies may be removed and sent to the laboratory to be analysed.

- There may be a small amount of bleeding following the procedure, but normal activities can be resumed immediately.

- If an abnormality is present, it may also be treated at this first visit.

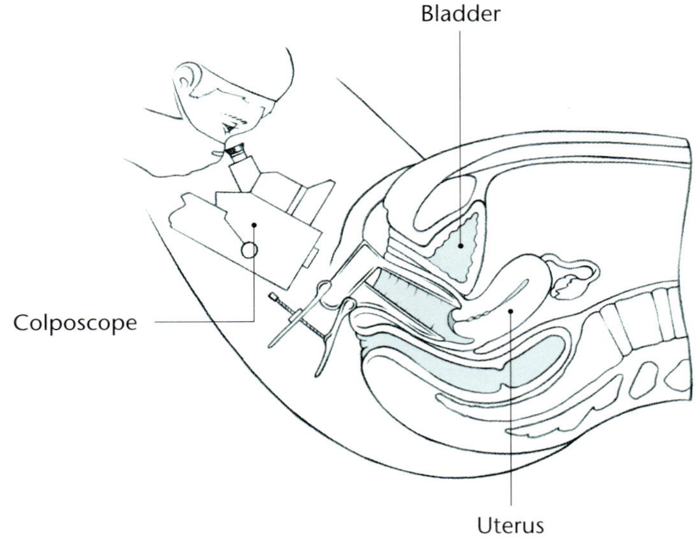

Bladder
Colposcope
Uterus

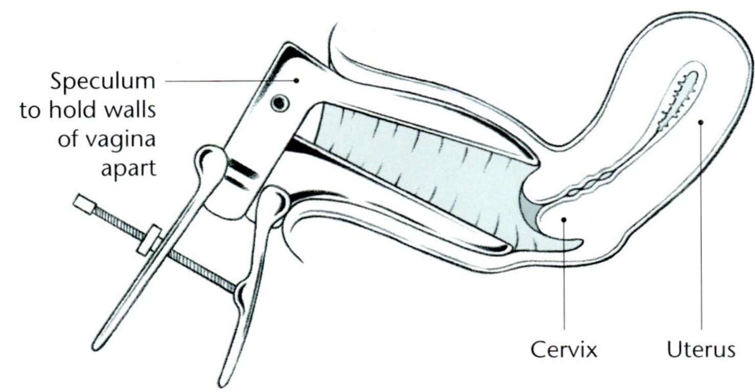

Speculum
to hold walls
of vagina
apart
Cervix
Uterus

Cone biopsy and cryocautery of the cervix

- Cone biopsy and cryocautery of the cervix are two methods used to remove abnormal cervical cells.

- Cone biopsy may be performed in out-patients under local anaesthetic or as a day-case operation in theatre under general anaesthetic. Cryocautery is a painless procedure carried out in out-patients.

- In both procedures, an instrument called a speculum is inserted to hold the walls of the vagina apart and the cervix is then examined with the colposcope. The colposcope is a microscope that magnifies the cervix and enables it to be seen more clearly.

- For a cone biopsy, the area to be removed is highlighted using iodine solution. A 'cone' of tissue, containing the abnormal area, is then removed using either a hot, wire loop or a laser. If performed in theatre, the tissue may be removed surgically and sent to the laboratory for examination.

- For cryocautery, the abnormal cells are destroyed by placing a freezing probe on the cervix for a few minutes.

- There may be some slight bleeding following these procedures. A vaginal discharge, which is dark brown or black in colour after cone biopsy, and light and clear after cryocautery, may also occur for up to 6 weeks. Any other discharge, particularly if offensive in smell, should be reported.

- Sexual intercourse should be avoided until after the next menstrual period to ensure that the cervix heals properly.

- Normal activities can be resumed the following day.

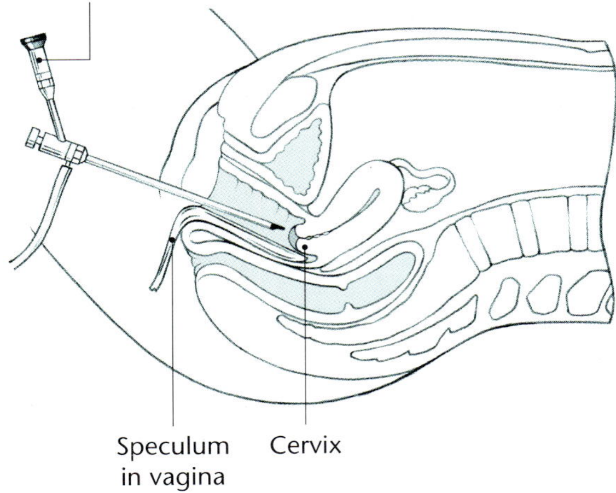

CONE BIOPSY

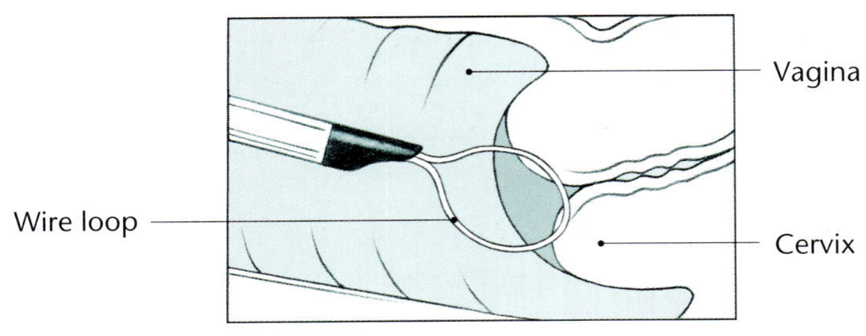

CRYOCAUTERY

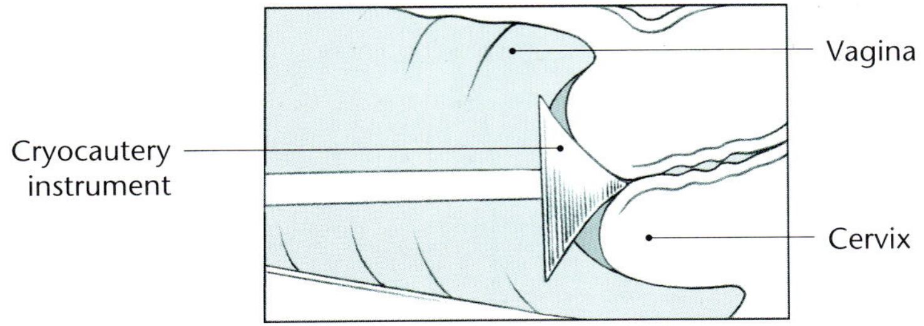

Radical hysterectomy

- Radical hysterectomy is used to treat some cases of cancer of the cervix. It involves removal of the uterus, Fallopian tubes, cervix, upper vagina, pelvic lymph glands and, occasionally, the ovaries. The vagina is stitched over at the top and shortened.

- The operation is performed under a general anaesthetic and takes 2–3 hours.

- During the operation, a catheter is passed up the urethra into the bladder to drain off the urine. A plastic tube may be inserted into the wound to remove any slight bleeding and fluid from the lymph glands. These tubes will be left in place for 24–48 hours.

- There will be some discomfort following surgery which will be controlled with pain killers, and hormone replacement therapy (HRT) may be prescribed if the ovaries are removed.

- The average hospital stay is 7–10 days. The time taken to make a full recovery varies and depends on many factors.

- Following surgery, a course of radiotherapy may be necessary.

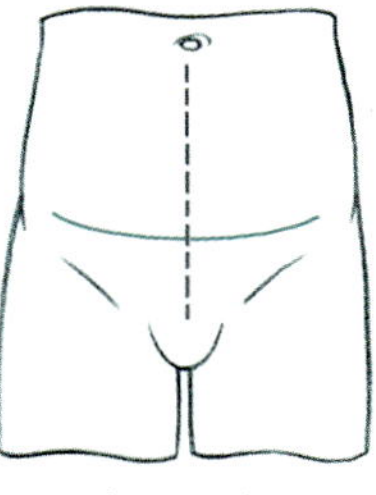

Alternative
incision sites

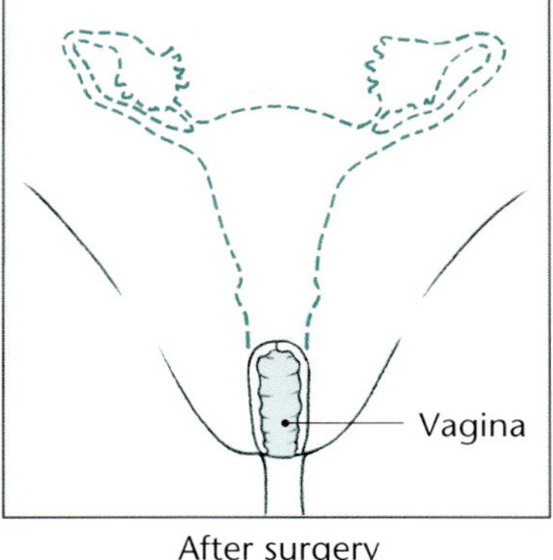

After surgery

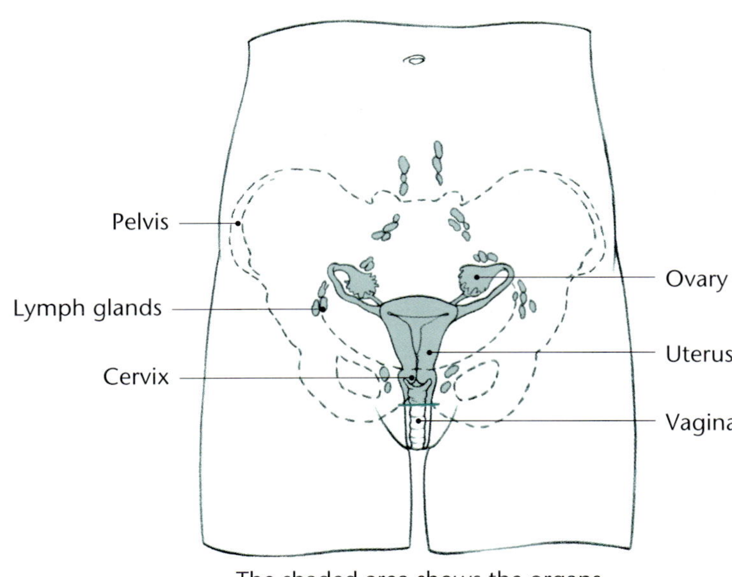

The shaded area shows the organs
that are removed

Ovarian tumour debulking

- Ovarian tumour debulking is a form of treatment for ovarian cancer. It involves removal of both ovaries, the uterus, cervix and omentum (fatty tissue overlying the bowel).

- The operation is performed under a general anaesthetic and may take several hours.

- Occasionally, a small portion of bowel affected by the cancer may need to be removed. This may result in a temporary (and rarely a permanent) stoma. A stoma is where the bowel opens directly onto the abdominal skin and faeces are collected in a bag attached to the abdominal wall.

- During the operation, a catheter is passed up the urethra into the bladder to drain off the urine. A plastic tube may be inserted into the wound to remove any slight bleeding. These tubes will be left in place for up to 72 hours.

- There will be some discomfort following surgery which will be controlled with pain killers.

- The average hospital stay is 14 days. The time taken to make a full recovery varies and depends on many factors.

- Following surgery, chemotherapy may be necessary.

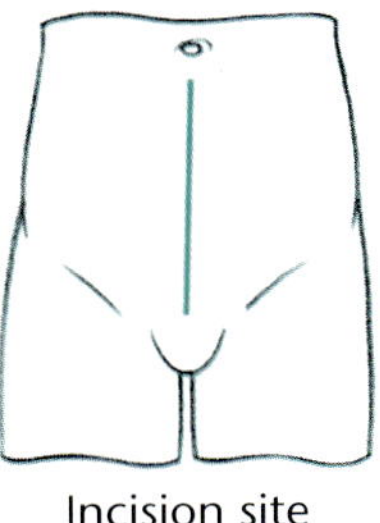

24

Incision site

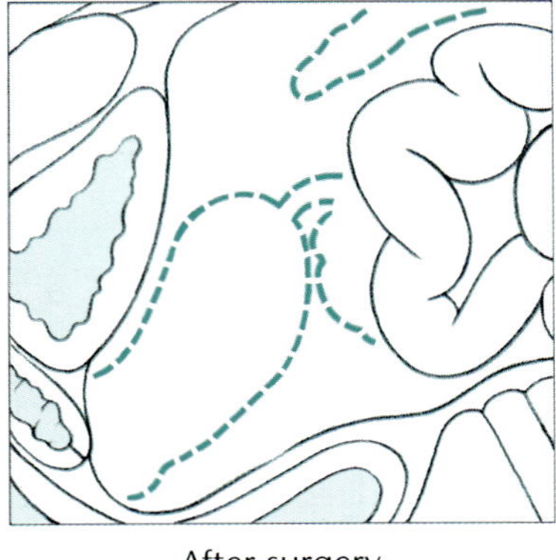

After surgery

The shaded area
shows the organs
that are removed

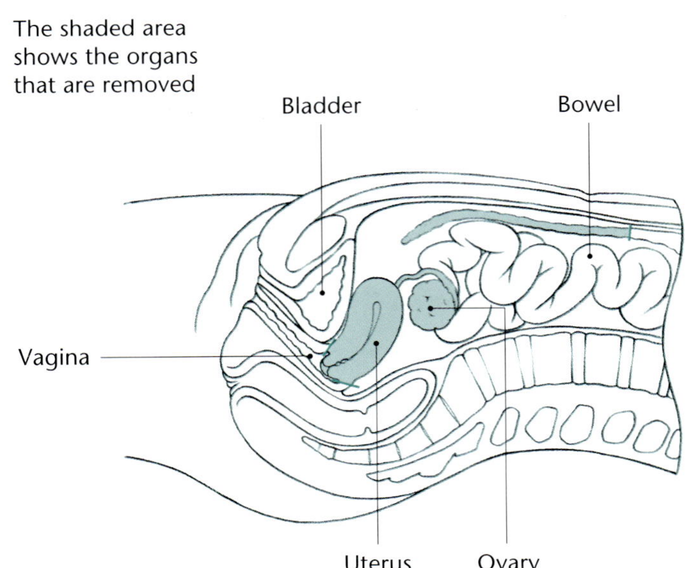

Vulvectomy and vestibulectomy

- A vulvectomy is used to treat skin conditions of the vulva only when other methods, such as creams, medicines and laser therapy, have failed. It involves removal of the vulva only. The urethra and vagina are left intact.

- A vestibulectomy is used to treat pain at the entrance to the vagina and is carried out only when other treatments have failed. It involves removal of the tissue at the entrance to the vagina.

- A partial vestibulectomy, which involves removal of only some of the tissue at the entrance to the vagina, may be used in conjunction with corticosteroid cream to treat a skin condition called lichen sclerosis.

- These operations are performed under a general anaesthetic and take 1–2 hours.

- In both operations, a catheter may be passed up the urethra into the bladder to drain off the urine. A plastic tube may also be inserted into the wound to remove any slight bleeding. These tubes will be left in place for up to 72 hours.

- There will be some discomfort following surgery which will be controlled with pain killers.

- The average hospital stay is 10–14 days and normal activities can usually be resumed within 6–8 weeks.

25

VULVECTOMY

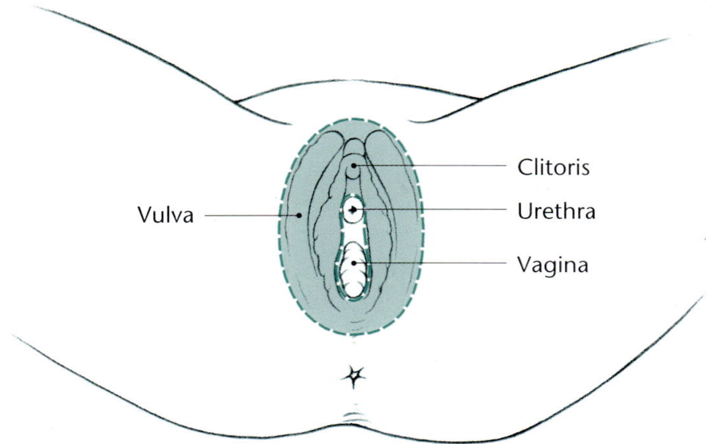

The shaded area shows the
organs that are removed

VESTIBULECTOMY

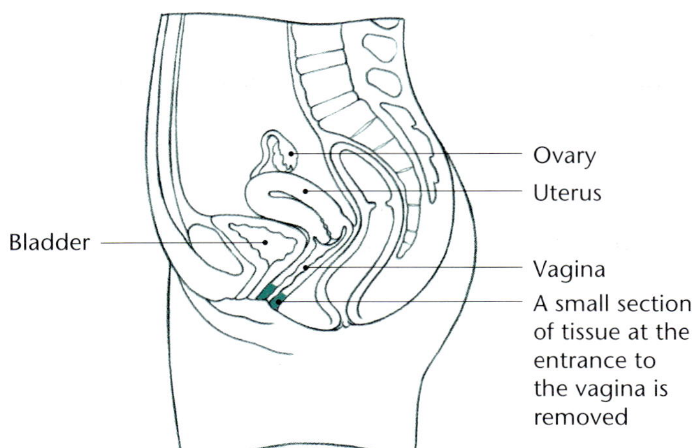

Radical vulvectomy

- Radical vulvectomy is used to treat cancer of the vulva. It involves removal of the vulva and the lymph glands in the groin. The urethra and vagina remain intact. Occasionally, skin grafting may be necessary to repair the wound.

- If the cancer has not spread to the sides of the vulva, around the clitoris, or between the vagina and anus, a simpler procedure can be carried out. This involves removal of only the skin around the cancer and the lymph glands in the groin.

- The operation is performed under a general anaesthetic and takes 2–3 hours.

- During the operation, a catheter is inserted into the bladder to drain off the urine. This may be brought out through the abdomen rather than the urethra to prevent irritation of the stitches. Two plastic tubes are also inserted to drain the fluid from the lymph glands. These tubes will be left in place for up to 72 hours.

- There will be some discomfort following surgery which will be controlled with pain killers.

- The average hospital stay is 2–3 weeks and normal activities can usually be resumed within 8–12 weeks.

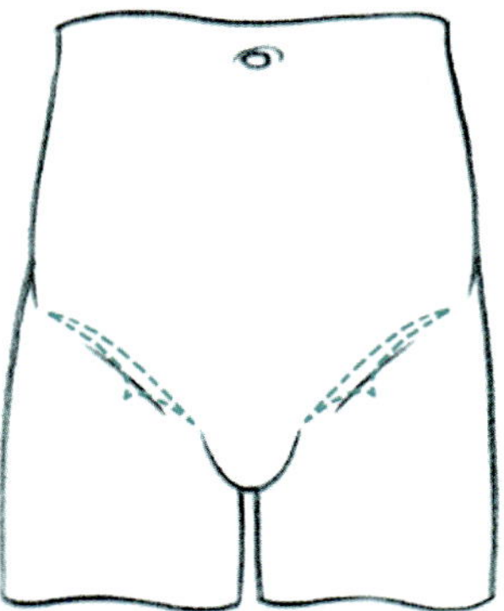

Incision sites for removal
of the lymph glands

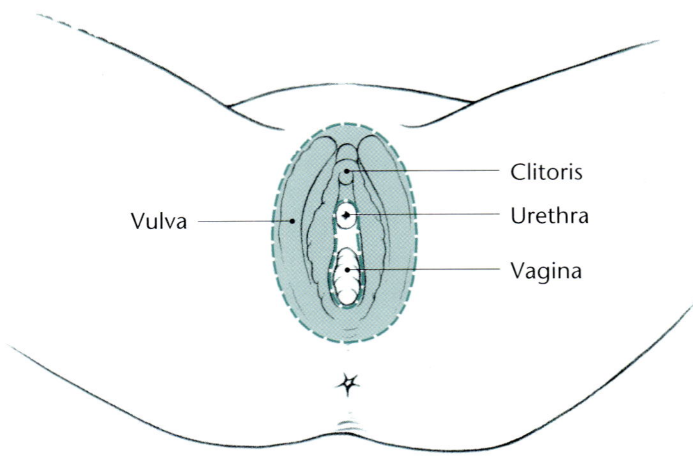

The shaded area shows the
organs that are removed

Vaginal hysterectomy and repair

- Vaginal hysterectomy and repair is the most commonly used operation to correct a prolapse or 'dropped' uterus caused by weakness in the muscles of the pelvic floor. Prolapse causes the uterus, bladder and sometimes the rectum (or back passage) to 'drop' through the vagina.

- In this operation, the uterus and cervix are removed through the vagina rather than through an abdominal incision. The bladder and rectum are also restored to their normal positions. The vagina is closed off and remains its normal length. The ovaries are left intact.

- The operation is carried out under a general anaesthetic and takes about $1-1\frac{1}{2}$ hours.

- During the operation, a catheter may be passed up the urethra into the bladder to drain off the urine. A vaginal pack made of gauze may also be inserted to prevent postoperative bleeding.

- There will be some discomfort following surgery which will be controlled with pain killers. Some postoperative bleeding and discharge should be expected.

- The average hospital stay is 4–5 days and normal activities can usually be resumed within 6 weeks.

BEFORE SURGERY

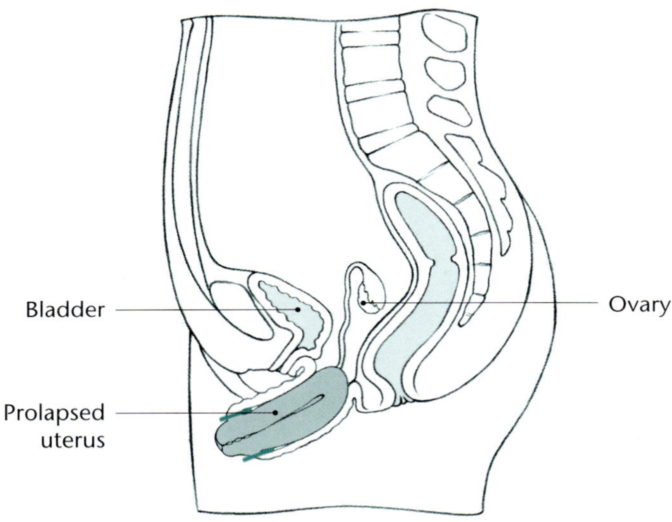

AFTER SURGERY

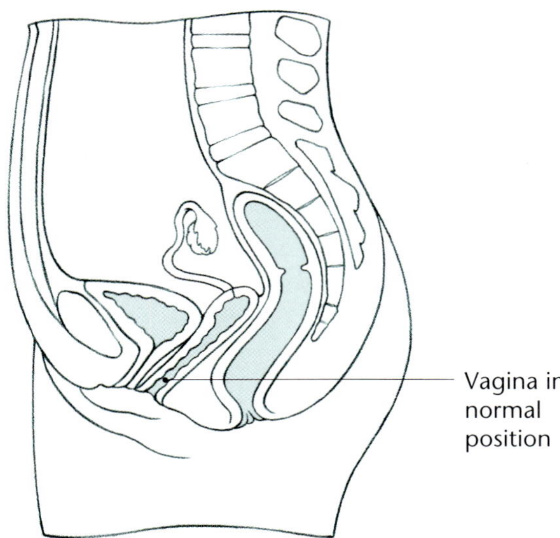

Prolapse repair (Manchester)

- The Manchester method of prolapse repair is performed to correct a prolapsed or 'dropped' uterus, caused by weakness in the muscles of the pelvic floor. Prolapse causes the uterus, bladder and sometimes the rectum (or back passage) to 'drop' through the vagina. This operation is performed only when the patient does not wish, or is not sufficiently fit, to have a vaginal hysterectomy.

- The operation is performed through the vagina. Only the cervix is removed. The uterus, bladder and rectum are stitched back into their normal positions.

- The operation is performed under a general anaesthetic and takes about 1 hour.

- During the operation, a catheter may be passed up the urethra into the bladder to drain off the urine. A vaginal pack made of gauze may also be inserted to prevent postoperative bleeding.

- There will be some discomfort following surgery which will be controlled with pain killers.

- The average hospital stay is 5–6 days and normal activities can usually be resumed within 6 weeks.

- Any subsequent pregnancy will have to be delivered by caesarean section to avoid stretching the previous repair.

BEFORE SURGERY

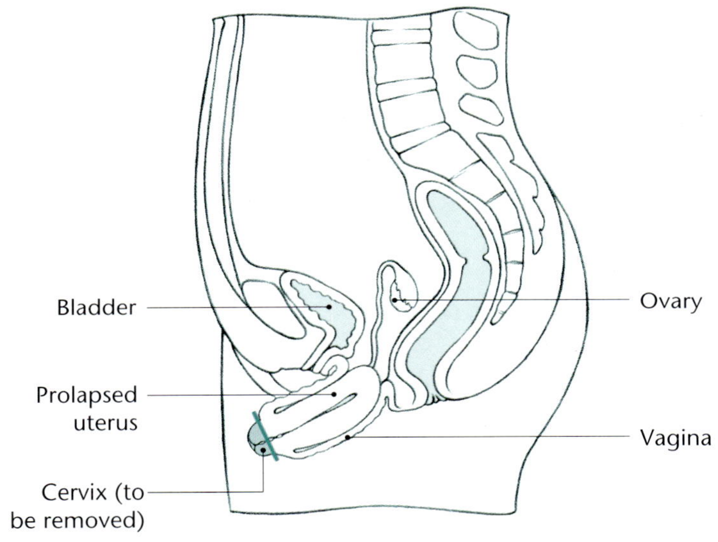

AFTER SURGERY

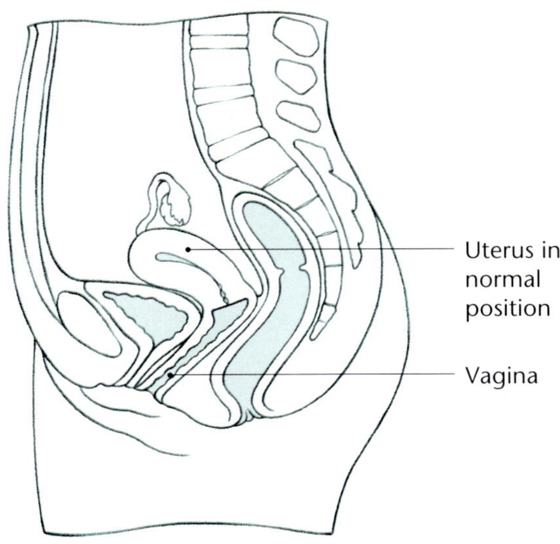

Ring pessary

- Insertion of a ring pessary is an alternative to surgery to correct a prolapsed or 'dropped' uterus caused by weakness in the muscles of the pelvic floor. Prolapse causes the uterus, bladder and sometimes the rectum (or back passage) to 'drop' through the vagina.

- This treatment is most suitable for patients who are not sufficiently fit to undergo a general anaesthetic or surgery.

- The ring pessary is a ring of plastic which is inserted into the vagina to support the bladder and uterus.

- Assessment and fitting are carried out in an out-patient clinic.

- The ring remains in the vagina, but must be changed every 6 months to prevent infection.

BEFORE INSERTION

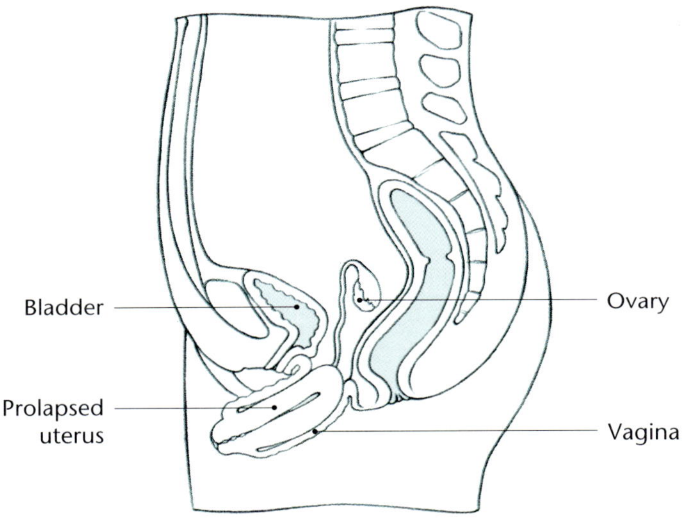

AFTER INSERTION

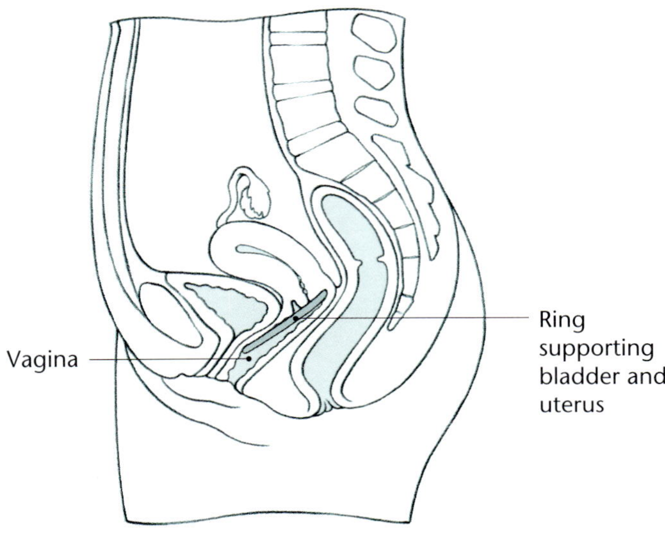

Cystocele (anterior) and rectocele (posterior) repair

- A cystocele occurs when the bladder and/or urethra prolapses or 'drops' into the front wall of the vagina. A rectocele occurs when the rectum prolapses or 'drops' into the back wall of the vagina.

- Repair involves removing a piece of vaginal skin, then stitching the bladder and urethra, or the rectum, back into their normal positions and repairing the vagina.

- Both types of repair and vaginal hysterectomy may be undertaken at the same time.

- The operation is carried out under a general anaesthetic and takes 40–60 minutes.

- During the operation, a catheter may be passed up the urethra into the bladder to drain off the urine. A vaginal pack made of gauze may also be inserted to prevent postoperative bleeding.

- There will be some discomfort following surgery which will be controlled with pain killers.

- The average hospital stay is 4–6 days and normal activities can usually be resumed within 6 weeks.

- The vagina may be left slightly narrowed, but this does not usually interfere with sexual intercourse.

CYSTOCELE

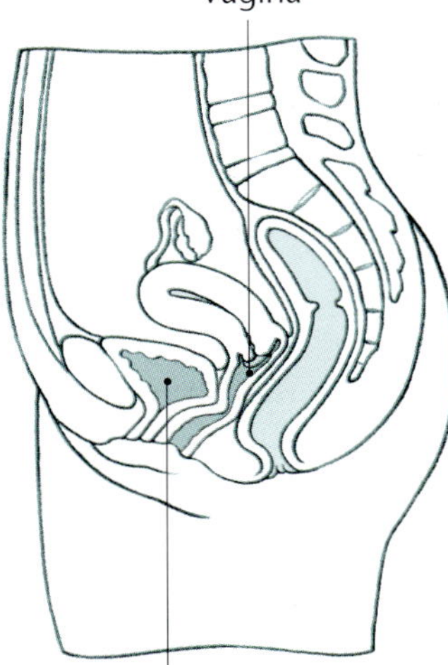

Before surgery, bladder prolapses into vagina

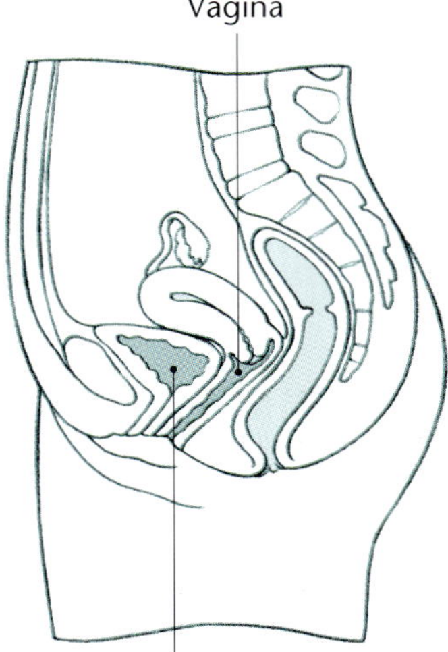

After surgery, normal position restored

RECTOCELE

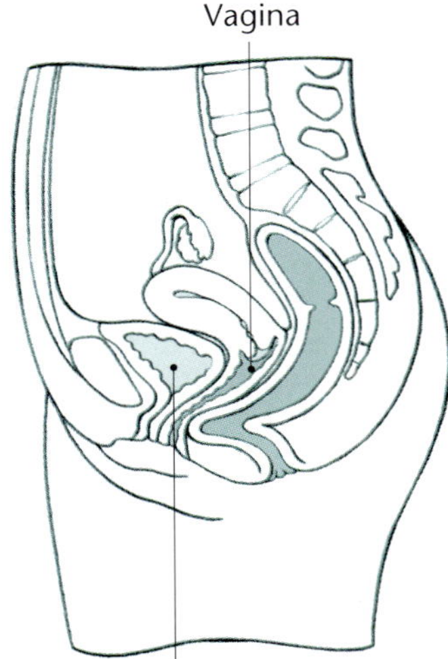

Before surgery, rectum prolapses into vagina

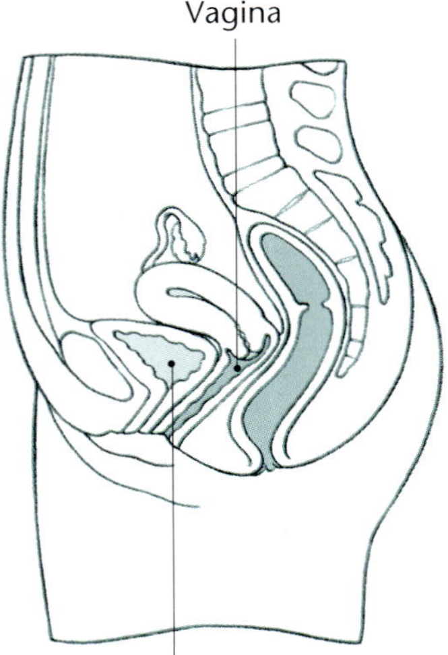

After surgery, normal position restored

Colposuspension

- Colposuspension is the ideal operation for urinary stress incontinence, which is caused by a weakness in the bladder neck and pelvic floor, usually as a result of pregnancy. Stitches are placed around the bladder neck in order to raise the bladder and urethra.

- The operation is performed under a general anaesthetic and takes 1–2 hours.

- During the operation, a catheter is inserted into the bladder to drain off the urine. This is usually brought out through the abdomen rather than the urethra.

- The catheter is 'clamped off' daily to allow the bladder to fill so that the patient can attempt to pass urine normally. If this is not possible, the clamp is released to drain the urine and the process repeated the following day. Once urine is being passed normally, the catheter is removed.

- There will be some discomfort following surgery which will be controlled with pain killers.

- The average hospital stay is 7–10 days and normal activities can usually be resumed within 6–8 weeks.

BEFORE SURGERY

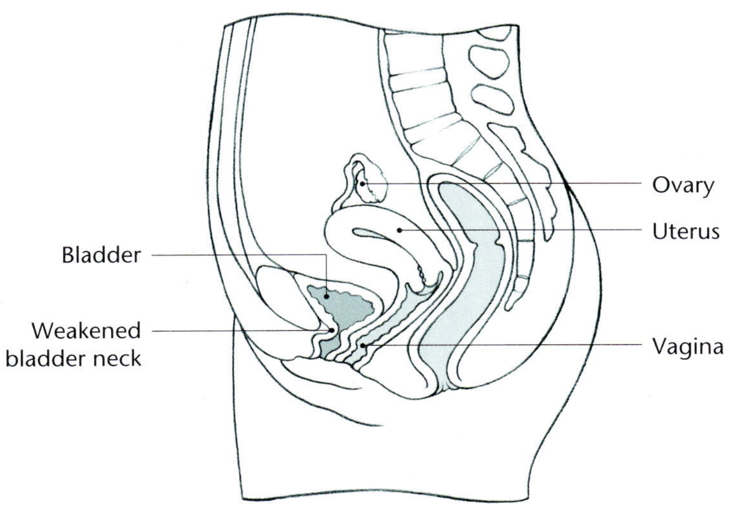

AFTER SURGERY

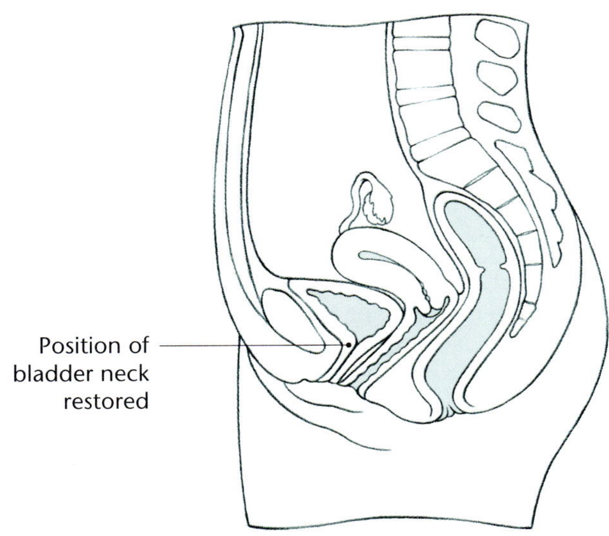

The menopause

- The menopause literally means the last menstrual period. The climacteric, which is commonly known as the menopause, is the time period in which symptoms occur, and oestrogen production falls and ultimately ceases.

- The menopause usually occurs between 48 and 52 years of age (the average in the UK is 51 years).

- Symptoms include hot flushes, sweats, psychological disturbances such as memory loss, concentration failure, depression and loss of libido, vaginal dryness, loss of bone density (osteoporosis), loss of breast tissue, skin thinning, discomfort during sexual intercourse, and urinary frequency and urgency. Irregular menstrual disturbances or sudden loss of menstruation may also occur.

- The symptoms can be treated with hormone replacement therapy (HRT). This may be either a combination of oestrogen and progesterone, or oestrogen alone if the patient has had a hysterectomy. HRT may be given as tablets, patches, implants or local vaginal preparations.

- With most HRT drugs, menstruation will continue until the woman stops taking the drug, but there are drugs that provide hormone replacement without causing bleeding.

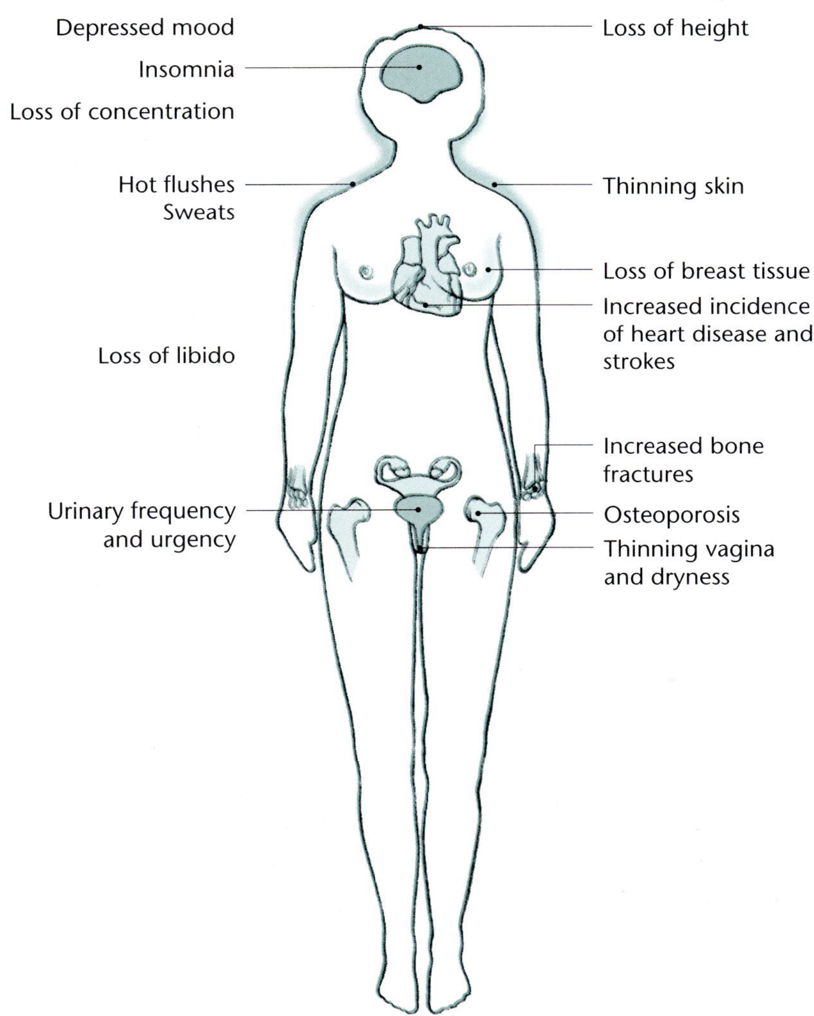
Depressed mood
Insomnia
Loss of concentration
Hot flushes
Sweats
Loss of libido
Urinary frequency
and urgency
Loss of height
Thinning skin
Loss of breast tissue
Increased incidence
of heart disease and
strokes
Increased bone
fractures
Osteoporosis
Thinning vagina
and dryness

Hormone replacement therapy – patches

- Patches may be used to provide hormone replacement therapy (HRT). Patches have the advantages that they give a more constant dose of hormone and require changing only once or twice a week.

- Patches may contain either a combination of oestrogen and progesterone, or oestrogen alone. If the uterus is still intact, a combination of oestrogen and progesterone is given, or an oestrogen-only patch with progesterone tablets for 2 weeks of the month. If the woman has previously undergone a hysterectomy, oestrogen is given alone.

- The patch is usually positioned on the lower body or thigh. It will need to be changed twice a week, but should not come off in the bath or when swimming.

- Irritation may occur, but this can be minimized if the patch is left open to the air for 1–2 minutes before being applied.

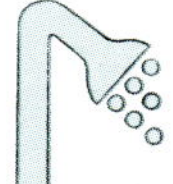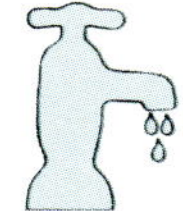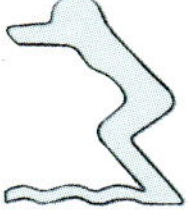

The patch should not come off during normal activities

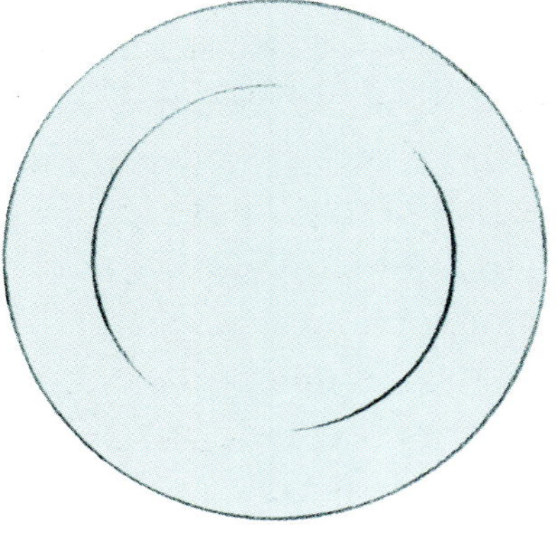

Actual size of patch

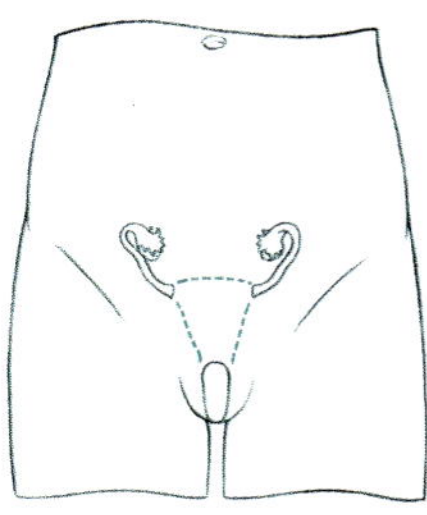

Patch contains only oestrogen if patient has had a hysterectomy

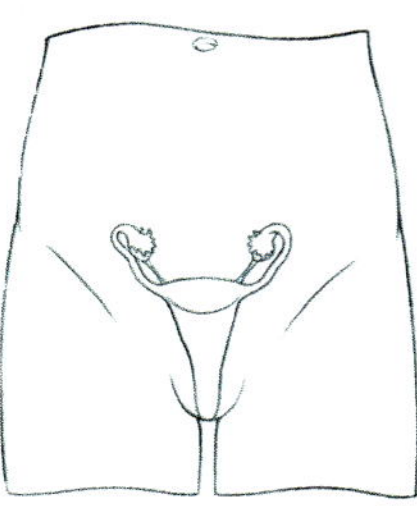

Patch contains oestrogen and progesterone if uterus is still present

Hormone replacement therapy – implants

- Implants may be used to provide hormone replacement therapy (HRT). Implants have the advantages that they give a more constant dose of hormone and need to be replaced only once every 6 months.

- Implants may contain oestrogen alone or a combination of oestrogen and testosterone. Testosterone is given if the woman is suffering loss of libido. Progesterone cannot be given as an implant and, if it is needed, must be given as tablets.

- Insertion of the implant is carried out under a local anaesthetic and takes about 5 minutes. The implant is inserted through a small incision about 1 centimetre long. The incision is then sometimes stitched at the end.

- Once in place, the implant cannot be removed, but will need to be replaced every 6 months.

- Usually, implants do not cause any problems and cannot be felt under the skin. Occasionally, however, an implant may be rejected and need to be reinserted.

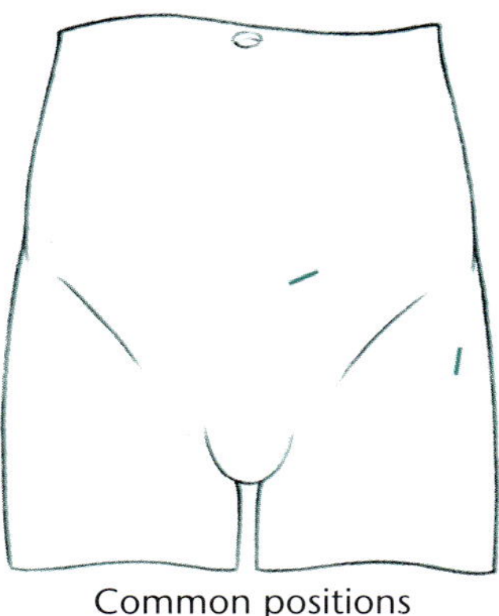

Common positions
for implant

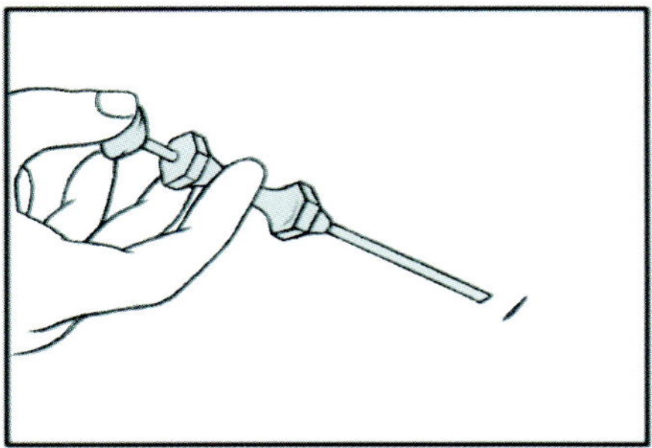

An introducer is used to insert the
implant through a small incision in
the skin

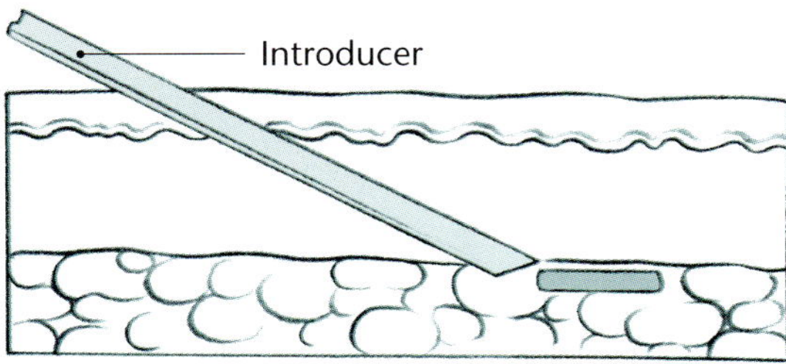

Implant lies in fat layer under skin

Mail Order

Additional copies of this book and other titles in the *Patient Pictures* series are available at a unit price of £10.95 (post-paid in the UK only).

Current titles include:
- Cardiology
- Fertility
- Gastroenterology
- Gynaecology
- HIV medicine
- Prostatic diseases and treatments
- Respiratory diseases
- Rheumatology
- Urological surgery

Please send your name and address, quantity required, and a cheque for the appropriate amount made payable to 'Health Press Limited' to:

Health Press Limited
Elizabeth House
Queen Street
Abingdon OX14 3JR

Health Press titles are available at special discounts when purchased in bulk quantities for trusts, associations or institutions. Please call our Special Sales Department in Abingdon on:

Tel: 01235 523233
Fax: 01235 523238